Doug Peterson's

SURVIVOR DIET CHALLENGE

volume 1

DISCLAIMER

I would be amiss if I did not suggest that you consult with your primary doctor before jumping head first into this challenge. So there you go. I am strongly suggesting that you do that. If you have some type of condition which may worsen under physical and mental stress then you may want to reconsider such a challenge. Or, if you think you might potentially develop some condition as a result of doing this challenge then perhaps this isn't for you.

That being said, I personally believe that the people who are apt to benefit most greatly from my Survivor Diet Challenge are the people who have the most extreme physical and mental deficiencies in all aspects of their lives. I just don't want to be held responsible if something should happen to someone as a result of taking on this challenge. So I am officially stating for the record that it is an individual choice to try my challenge and I am not responsible for anything negative that might happen as a result of someone attempting it. If you attempt this, you are on your own.

CONTENTS

FORWARD

In the time line of human existence, we've been eating food that we've hunted, grown, or gathered for more than 200,000 years. Our bodies have evolved in accordance to the food we ate and the lifestyles we lived. We hunted, fished, trapped small animals, and gathered fruit, tubers, leaves and seeds. We ate most of the foods within days, usually hours. Our hunter-gatherer ancestors ate more than one hundred species of plants, rich in vitamins, fiber and nutrients. They ate a large variety of animals including large game, rodents and even termites and grubs. This variety of food guaranteed a range of nutrients we can't come close to today. Genetically, we are the same as our hunter-gatherer ancestors, but our worlds are vastly different.

There's no point in repeating the statistics of obesity and diseases that have developed in recent history as a result of our food and lifestyle choices as we've gained more and more distance from our hunter-gatherer ancestors. It's been drilled into our modern heads again and again that we need to eat more vegetables, less meat, little sugar, and get off our butts and exercise. We know to do these things, but we still don't do them. It's too easy and delicious not to. Bring a caveman from 20,000 years ago into present time and he, too, would end up on the couch eating pizza and ice cream.

We are all hostages of modern convenience delivered to us by our own trusted government through the USDA, who promoted eating from the food guide pyramid that told us to gorge on pasta and bread, meat and cheese. Our overweight, diseased bodies have the government and their lobbyists to thank for providing sugar-laden, artificially flavored and colored food-like items to fill the eye-level shelves of our local supermarkets. They approved of their colorful and convincing messages telling us of their generous nutrients and delicious flavors, despite not being entirely true. And they train professionals to say that to gain back health, patients should eat lower fat, but artificially sweetened and artificially flavored food-like items. It's no wonder that people have lost touch with their senses and don't have any idea of what eating real food means.

But there are those who were never fooled by the USDA or their lobbyists, and have been fighting a revolution for decades against fake foods. Though they are in the minority, they've still planted seeds in the ears of many, and the message of real food seems to be gaining ground.

One of those seeds has sprouted in the ear of Doug Peterson, my husband, after years and years of my ranting. Of course, he couldn't go about his health quest my way. It just isn't in him to be a follower. Besides, it's just plain boring to simply change your diet and habits by following a nutrition counselor's guidance. He had to do it his own way, and he had to make it an adventure. And so he did.

The transformation he undertook over those first 40 days was truly amazing. He went from a moody, lazy, uninspired, lump on the couch (with a pot belly) to a slimmed-down, energetic, dynamic and driven man. And he was down-right sexy. Of course, it wasn't all glamorous. He had low points when the weather didn't cooperate or he didn't have the time to hunt or gather his food for that day. But, that only inspired him to plan better and figure out how to get through the lean days. By the third week, he was feeling better than ever and would wonder, out loud why he ever ate food that wasn't real.

Before his Survivor Diet Challenge, he would be sluggish during the day, snore during the night, have migraine headaches regularly, as well as gas and bloating. During his SDC this all went away. His doctor, who previously told him he'd need to go on several medications, actually began to re-think some of his treatment methods.

Though he did it for no one but himself, I've used Doug's SDC story countless times with my clients, trying to convince them that eating real food is what our bodies need to heal, and that all our genetically hunter-gatherer bodies want is for us to get off our butts and eat foods that don't have labels or come in boxes, bags or packages of any kind. His story has inspired hundreds of people, not necessarily to take on his challenge, but to follow its premise.

Our bodies have evolved over millennia to become the fine machine it is, constantly doing all it can do to maintain homeostasis. Its natural state is health, and so it will be if we fuel it with what it needs. Our hunter-gatherer ancestors had no other choice than to eat the right things. Unfortunately, our modern way, so wonderful for the most part, is also what's killing us painfully by taking us further away from our true selves. I challenge you to get back to what your body is designed to be, whether it's following advice like mine to eat real food and live a healthier lifestyle within the world you've created or to have a grand adventure trying Doug's Survivor Diet Challenge. Either way, you'll feel better than ever. So, what are you waiting for?

Debbie Peterson, MA, CHC

PREFACE

The human being is a remarkable self-sustaining, self-repairing organic machine. It is capable of truly amazing things and we have only begun to scratch the surface of understanding its boundless potential.

We all own one of these machines. And despite our continual efforts to breakdown and destroy our machines over a lifetime, they keep bouncing back. They keep rebuilding. Healing. Our machines grow and get stronger and even get smarter. They continually learn as we bombard them with new challenges and new experiences year after year.

Despite diseases, viruses, bacterial invaders, physical injuries – all stresses that we deal with over a lifetime, our machine, our body, figures out how to defend against them and continues to thrive. More powerful than a super computer, the repair system of our body works feverishly day and night without rest. All we have to do to maintain this miraculous piece of equipment is to feed it the fuel that it needs. But what do we do instead? We feed it poison. Poison in the form of fast food, junk food, preservatives, genetically modified organisms, chemicals, artificial colors and flavoring, etc. - all disguised as real food fuel.

We aren't intentionally trying to kill our body by feeding it poison. After all, our minds have been tricked into thinking it is actually food. It looks like food. It tastes and smells like food. So what is it? Over the years, we have become desensitized to the evolution of our food. Time has allowed food to trick us as it has been slowly transforming.

In a worldwide effort to make our body's fuel more accessible and more convenient to acquire, we have been changing it - modifying what once was actual food. In an attempt to improve it, we have actually turned it against us. You know the stuff I'm talking about. It's everywhere. All of a sudden, in the evolutionary blink of an eye, the modified foodstuff is all around us – inescapable. It is engineered to last longer, taste better, to be more addicting and alluring and to be "healthier" than ever - a grandiose deception.

We are also transforming. After all, you are what you eat – right? Despite the poisoning of our machines, our bodies are still able to adapt and go on. The machines adapt and change to use the new fuel but the changes do not come without a price. The adaptations are ugly - distorted mutations of what our machines are supposed to be. At some point even these remarkable, self-repairing machines will no longer be able to rebound or take the abuse.

Who is to blame for this ruse? Who can we point the finger at and hold accountable? Big Business certainly plays its part. The almighty dollar is filling the pockets of a few, through the contributions of many who would pay for a more convenient fuel source. After all, we are busy little machines – always on the go, go, go. Time is a valuable commodity. If we can minimally get through the day with the body fuel that is readily accessible and all around us, then we will pay a premium for it. We pay for the convenience. As this type of fuel becomes more and more popular, Big Business will make more and more of it – and the price will drop lower and lower. How easy is that?

In defense of Big Business, they are also doing their part to make our body fuel more accessible and more convenient worldwide. Wait a minute. That sounds like the same reason why we are blaming them and why we are holding them partially accountable for this deception! Well, essentially it is. While Big Business is fattening its pockets, it has also played an important positive role in contributing to the evolution and development of our civilization today.

As populations grow, finding a dependable source of food fuel for our machines becomes increasingly difficult. The fuel needs to be made available and on a much, much larger scale. It needs to be imported from here, exported to there, shipped, flown, distributed and delivered to wherever it is needed the most. Only Big Business could accomplish such an enormous undertaking. And without Big Business, our society would not have been able to grow to what it has become today. It helps to fulfill a need. You can choose to look at Big Business in a negative light when it comes down to the food fuel that it produces. But, its contributions to our human civilization cannot be overlooked. Its original intentions were to help solve a problem – How to keep the machines running? How to keep us alive and help us grow and prosper and explore and expand?

Big Business just could not see, over the course of so many years, that the food fuel began to transform. It didn't happen overnight. These changes occur very gradually over the course of hundreds of years – or more. The change is almost imperceptible. Our machines started to notice though. After a while the machines began to break down. They got slower, less efficient and problems that were previously repairable were not so easily repaired.

Some people are forced to change their food fuel because of illness or disease or intolerance to certain things that their body just cannot cope with. More and more we hear terms like peanut allergies, lactose intolerance, gluten free and many others. Have these things always been a part of our culture? Or are they becoming more and more prevalent as changes to our foods continue to evolve and transform? It is difficult to tell when the changes happen so slowly – imperceptibly.

A few strong people have figured it out and have made a conscious decision to go against the common trend. Terms like holistic, healthy, organic, earthy/crunchy and others represent a slowly growing minority of people who are looking at the fuel for their machines in a different light. They have begun to question the popular belief. It takes strength of character and conviction to question what is commonly accepted and to pave a new path for yourself, for your machine. To pave a new future.

I don't claim to have all of the answers but I am courageous enough to ask the questions and to try to make changes in order to grow and prosper. The following pages will chronicle my personal experiences through my self-imposed culinary challenge – a vision quest if you will. Come along on my journey as I attempt to change the world, one person at a time. Perhaps some of it will enlighten and inspire you to make similar changes within yourself and to spread the information to others. It's time to get our machines working properly again.

"It's ok not to know all the answers. It's better to admit our ignorance than to believe answers that might be wrong. Pretending to know everything closes the door to finding out what's really there."
~Neil deGrasse Tyson

INTRODUCTION

Last year I had quite a lazy winter. I had reconstructive surgery on my knee which kept me bound to my living room couch for quite some time. With very little exercise and lots of eating, I started to feel like crap. I was getting headaches regularly, my blood pressure was considerably high and after every meal my stomach just had this full and bloated feeling that didn't go away. I had trouble sleeping, with restless and uncomfortable nights and periodic bouts of snoring that didn't go over very well with my wife. Does any of that sound familiar?

Something prompted me to go to my doctor for a physical and the first thing he did was put me on the scale. It read 200 pounds! I laughed and told him that his scale was off by about 10 pounds. I had been weighing myself regularly and the most I ever weighed at home was 190. He laughed back and proceeded to go into detail about how his professionally calibrated scale was NOT off. The rest of the visit went the same way – me challenging the quality of his blood pressure monitoring equipment - followed by detailed explanations as to the validity of his diagnostic tests. Etc, etc. After my denial phase, I finally realized that something needed to change. Guess what he suggested? That's right - diet and exercise! Two words that, until then, had never been part of my vocabulary.

Knowing myself better than my doctor, I immediately knew that I would most certainly not conform to the "normal" weight loss diet or the typical gym member's regular exercise routines. Faced with this dilemma I asked myself a very important question: **How can I lose weight and get healthy without traditional dieting or exercise and have fun and adventure in the process?** I knew that if I could somehow link a weight loss program to having fun and adventure then there was a chance I could make it work.

The answer . . . my "Survivor Diet Challenge"

The answer came to me one evening while sitting on my couch watching television (ironic). I was watching an episode of my favorite 'Reality TV' show, appropriately named *Survivor*. Anyone who has watched this popular show knows that the contestants who actually survive to the end

(40 days) usually end up weighing and looking like a fraction of their original selves. If you haven't seen the show, the basic premise is that a group of people are dropped off on a remote tropical island and must use their wit and survival skills to outlast the other contestants. They are forced back to their primal roots and must learn to find their own food to survive. They are usually provided with a basic ration of rice and beans as well as a water supply at the start. Occasionally, throughout the 40 day time period, they compete in reward challenges and the winners are either given something special to eat or are provided with a tactical survival advantage.

When I watch the show I can't help think to myself how much fun it would be. Sure, the winner of the show gets a large cash prize but even without the prize it seems like it would be an experience of a lifetime. There is excitement and adventure and intrigue around every corner, every day. For 40 days, they sure do get their exercise. And as far as diet, well, that depends on the skills of the individuals. Season after season, one common trend remains – all the contestants lose a significant amount of weight after 40 days.

So, this is how my Survivor Diet Challenge was born and accompanying the challenge comes a set of rules and guidelines to adhere to. For 40 days I will live off the land. I will pick, gather, hunt, collect, dig, and catch whatever I can find to eat. I will give myself a ration of rice and beans at the beginning as well as an unlimited supply of water. Occasionally I will reward myself for accomplishments but I will stick to the guidelines to the best of my ability.

Not everyone is cut out for my Survivor Diet Challenge. There are people with certain skill sets and personality types that will see this as a true challenge and welcome the unique and interesting experience that will ensue. Yet there are others who will be adamantly against the whole premise – as with anything new and different I suppose. If you think my Survivor Diet Challenge is for you, feel free to take it on and share your experiences with others. You can use my general rules and guidelines as a starting point but feel free to customize and write your own rules based on your personal circumstances.

Try not to stray too far from the original set of rules. Much time and thought went into their creation and if this challenge catches on like I think it may, it would be nice if everyone had the same standards. Also, try the best you can not to 'cheat' or stray too far from the terms of the diet during this challenge. It only hurts you in the long run. Make a list of cheats whenever you stray so that you can be honest with yourself and possibly trade future rewards for moments of weakness.

One thing I promise is that you will learn a great deal, stay very busy and active, have a lot of fun, suffer and struggle a bit – and in the end you will have a tremendous life experience and many stories of your own to tell.

Rules and Official Guidelines

The duration of the challenge is 40 days. The rules are quite simple:

- You must survive on only the food that you can grow, find or catch outdoors.

- You can have as much water as you want.

- You can cook with your own stove, microwave, grill, etc. and use whatever pots, pans, dishes, refrigerator, etc. that you need.

- You may also use whatever resources you have in order to obtain your food. For example, if you are trying to catch fish you can use whatever fishing equipment you have – or you may purchase any fishing equipment or tackle necessary – including bait (but you can't eat the bait!).

- You will provide yourself with a gallon container allotment each of beans and brown rice at the start. You will be responsible to ration these items appropriately throughout the 40 days. Eat too much at the start and you will be left with very little at the end.

- As a bonus, you will be granted periodic rewards to celebrate each full week of successful completion of the challenge.

- If you work a full work week, here's an (optional) added bonus: One time per week you are allowed to have a complete sushi lunch. I chose sushi because not only is it delicious and nutritious, but it is probably the closest thing to survivor food – so enjoy one lunch per week but don't take advantage of this by going overboard.

WEEKLY REWARDS

- After Week 1 you may reward yourself with one pound of butter and a container of pepper corns. Make it last! This will help to spice up and flavor your foods.

- After Week 2 you may reward yourself with flour, bread crumbs and vegetable oil. Well done - at the two week mark you may have some fish to bread and fry. Be creative. There may be some other uses for these reward items.

- After Week 3 you may reward yourself with fruit: one orange, one lemon and one whole pineapple. The sweetness of these fruits will give you a boost – not to mention the vitamin C. Well done. See how long you can make them last.

- After Week 4 you may reward yourself with. . . MEGABURGER! Go find the biggest, baddest, burger you can possibly imagine - with all the fixings. Add some fries and a big ol' beer if you'd like. Make this a treat to look forward to and one to remember.

- After Week 5 you may reward yourself with a meal of your choosing - ANYTHING! Treat yourself - you deserve it for surviving 5 weeks. Maybe try making a suckling pig (just a thought) or something exotic that you've never had before.
  Hang in there – almost finished!

SPECIAL OCCASION REWARDS

Occasionally, throughout the course of this diet you may take part in "Special Occasion" activities. Examples of these include birthday parties, holidays, celebratory barbecues, etc. When you find yourself in these Special Occasion situations you have a choice to make. You can stay the course and continue with the Survivor Diet, or you can choose to invoke a "Special Occasion Reward." When you do this, you can take part in that special occasion but in exchange, you must give up one of your weekly rewards. It can be one you've already earned (except for something already eaten), or a future reward.

HEALTHOMETER

Is the Survivor Diet healthy? This question has been brought to the forefront on several occasions. How do you determine the relative 'health' of an individual? After all, it is sometimes a difficult subject to measure and quantify.

Obviously, weight should be measured and closely monitored on a daily basis. This will be one piece of the puzzle. Another relatively easy thing to measure is blood pressure. Going in, I have known that I have a moderately high blood pressure after visiting my doctor. We will see if a dramatic change in diet and weight will have any effect on blood pressure as I progress through the challenge.

Another symptom of ill-health that I have been experiencing on a somewhat regular basis is the presence of migraine headaches. Although difficult to measure, I will keep a close watch on the relationship between headaches and dietary changes and report my findings.

I thought about having a complete physical with full blood test done before and after the diet. This would be another way to try to quantify the results to see if there were any beneficial or detrimental changes as a result of such an extreme diet. I did not follow through with this testing but I will certainly consider doing this in the future if the Survivor Diet becomes an annual event. It would be nice to have some concrete documentation to substantiate changes in health whether they are good or bad.

We know that obesity is linked to a variety of other illness and disorders that afflict our society today such as diabetes, coronary heart disease, high blood pressure, stroke, cancers, sleeping disorders, to name a few. By reducing overall weight, is it accurate to say that the potential risk for all of these other conditions will also be reduced? In the upcoming weeks I will be pondering this link and logging any noticeable changes in my health. Perhaps I will identify some connection.

In addition to the underlying goal of losing weight, my Survivor Diet will hopefully act as a means to detoxify and cleanse my system over the course of 40 days. When I think about all of the unnatural chemicals and preservatives that are incorporated into our industrially processed foods these days, I can't help but believe that my body is going to welcome such a change. This too will certainly have an overall health impact. It may be difficult to measure but perhaps there is a way or a sign that presents itself during the course of the challenge.

In the future I may have more knowledge and information that will open doors to other tests and means to track changes in overall health. For now, my daily Healthometer log which tracks changes in weight and blood pressure will have to suffice.

Keep a log of your own experiences during this challenge. It gets interesting. A log is an important part of the learning process. Having something to look back on can help in so many ways. Learn from mistakes and re-live your successes because you kept a log. It also helps to reveal trends which otherwise may have gone unnoticed. Certain foods may be triggering headaches while others may give you stomach pains. Use your log and the scientific method to analyze trends in your dietary habits and come to your own conclusions about which foods give you the most significant health benefits.

Preparation for the Challenge

If you are considering creating your own Survivor Diet Challenge or closely following mine, there are some things to consider before jumping right into it. Some planning and preparation is always good, but there is also a certain degree of the unknown which needs to be explored through trial and error and personal experience.

The start and end dates of your challenge should be determined based on the climate and seasons of the particular region in which you live. I can only tell you why I chose the dates I selected for my challenge and you will have to use your common sense in order to derive your own.

I live in New Jersey and I live on the East coast very close to the ocean. For me, the winter is a time of cold, lifeless, solitude. Nature is in hibernation mode. Toward the end of March and April the signs of spring are very apparent all around us. Warmth and color return to the area and with it brings a whole migration of living creatures. It's the cycle of life. This is a time when I am anxious to get active again outdoors. I have been cooped up all winter and it is time to bust out. For me, this is the perfect time to start my 40 day challenge.

I also have to consider the timing of other potential food sources like growing vegetables in a garden or seasonal restrictions to hunting or fishing for certain animal species. Some of these seasons intersect with each other yet others will not be available until mid to late summer. Depending on what my needs for the challenge may be, I will decide on the start and end dates so that I can maximize the availability of a variety of well-liked food sources. I suggest that you take your home area into consideration in a similar way and do the same. The dates that work for me in New Jersey will most likely not work for someone in Australia.

The next thing that I would consider is your overall health condition. I would be amiss if I did not suggest that you consult with your primary doctor before jumping head first into the challenge. So there you go. I am strongly suggesting that you do that. If you have some type of condition which may worsen under physical and mental stress then you may want to reconsider such a challenge. Or, if you think you might potentially develop some condition as a result of the same stress to your system then perhaps this isn't for you.

That being said, I personally believe that the people who are apt to benefit most greatly from my Survivor Diet Challenge are the people who have the most extreme physical and mental deficiencies in all aspects of their lives. I just don't want to be held responsible if something should happen to someone as a result of taking on this challenge. So I am officially stating for the record that it is an individual choice to try my challenge and I am not responsible for anything negative that might happen as a result of someone attempting it. If you attempt this, you are on your own. That should be enough of a disclaimer.

Something that I found helpful while on this diet was to tell my co-workers, friends and family all about it. When I began I was a bit secretive - thinking people would make fun of such an extreme diet. What was more difficult was eating strange lunches at work and rejecting treats and other 'normal' offerings from people. That made me seem strange until I finally came out of the closet and revealed my purpose and my reasons for behaving strangely. Once people understand that you are trying to do something new and different to hopefully improve your health and well-being, they will be very supportive. In fact, you will find that people will then start to help you in your quest to find new sources of food. So by all means, put it out there right from the start. Don't try to hide it because it will be very obvious to the people closest to you that something different is going on in your life. Embrace and welcome the support of others and perhaps you will influence someone else to make positive changes in their life.

Other things necessary to prepare for this challenge can be learned along the way. It would be helpful if you have some prior survival skill sets but learning and acquiring these skills is also part of the challenge. Learn by trying and doing and experimenting. Make mistakes. Have fun and have a great adventure.

That's it. Can you survive my Survivor Diet Challenge?

Good luck.

Prequel and Acknowledgments

My very first, original Survivor Diet Challenge was in 2009. At the time, the Survivor Diet was just a simple idea without rules, guidelines or rewards. It was a 40 day experiment without a name and was somewhat disorganized. I did not keep a log or a journal of my daily activities but I do remember wishing that I had. After it was over I told myself that if I should ever do this again I will organize it and document it every step of the way. I could immediately tell that this was something special and something that others might enjoy as well. Through my words and experiences, I hoped to inspire anyone who was willing and able to take on their own Survivor Diet Challenge.

The following pages are the actual daily accounts of my Survivor Diet Challenge in 2010. That is why, from time to time, you may read references to "the first time I did this" or "last year's Survivor Diet." This is the first time I attempted to document my adventures with both written words and photographs – and I also experimented a bit with some videography – which may become a larger part in future challenges.

I would also like to take this opportunity to thank my family who helped me out every step of the way - especially when my will power was faltering. My wife, Debbie who is a certified health and nutrition counselor, has been ultra supportive despite my odd behaviors at times. My kids, Ty and Jamie have really enjoyed sharing in my adventures and in several cases have over-enjoyed sharing in my meals. At the onset of this challenge they were nine and seven years old, respectively, and I truly believe that some of our activities will be remembered and reminisced for a lifetime.

DAY 1 - THE BEGINNING (APRIL 12, 2010)

"Only those who dare to fail greatly can ever achieve greatly."
~Robert F. Kennedy

Well, here we go. This is the official start to my Survivor Diet Challenge of 2010. It will hopefully run from April 12th through May 21st - ending on Memorial Day weekend.

Each day I am planning on waking up and recording my weight and blood pressure and at some point in the morning I will take a photo from the belly up and a profile photo.

Today I was excited to get started but I have to say that I was a little nervous about what I was about to embark upon.

Hmmm . . . What's for breakfast?

My agenda for today was to get my rations of beans and rice and some containers to put them in. I also have to get some greens from the lawn and I have a great idea for some seasonings. I have been trying to find some places to catch fish for the past couple of days but have been unsuccessful. I am a little worried about that.

We are in the heart of winter flounder season, trout season officially opened two days ago, and there have been great striped bass reports online lately. However, I got skunked opening day and the next day for trout, and yesterday I tried for some flounder in the Shrewsbury River for a few hours without even a bite! I should have gone striper fishing on a charter boat today because of the reports, but I didn't get up early enough and the party boats are already gone. I guess I'll work on some protein later.

I went to Whole Foods™ and stocked up on red/white kidney beans and short grain brown rice. I got about a gallon of each. Then I went to Bed Bath and Beyond for a couple of gallon sized, plastic containers to store my rations.

After that I took a ride to the beach to see if there were any signs of fish to be caught. It was beautiful outside but the ocean was like a desert. No signs of life anywhere. No boats as far as I could see - nobody fishing.

So I bagged the idea of catching any fish and decided to work on my spices. Last year when I did the Survivor Diet Challenge I gave myself some spices as a reward after the first week. Salt, in particular was a very welcome addition to my meals. It's amazing how much you miss salt after not having it. This year I had the idea to get my salt from the most abundant source of salt on the planet - the ocean!

I brought a five gallon bucket with me to the beach but I didn't bring my waders and I didn't want to get all wet trying to fill my bucket with water in the waves. I didn't have any rope either. I walked out the end of a rock jetty and saw a place I could dip the bucket, but it was a little out of reach and the rocks down by the waterline were dangerously slippery. I searched for some rope and eventually found some old washed up rope between some of the rocks. It wasn't very long so I had to untwist the strands and tie them together at the ends to make one long rope that I could use to get my water. After a couple tries I was successful and I brought my bucket full of ocean water back home.

I filtered the water by straining it through a couple layers of t-shirts, put it into a big stainless steel pot and onto the stove top. I'll make a long story short here - I boiled the water down (took all day long, finished at 11pm) and what I was left with was about a cup and a half of pure white, sea salt. Success! That should last me quite a while. And if I ever need more . . . it will be very easy to repeat the process.

Ok - protein. Last year, when the fishing wasn't so good, clams became my main meals in the beginning. I had to drop Jamie off at gymnastics at 4:30 and low tide at my clam spot was at about 2:30. She has gymnastics for two hours and my spot is about 15 minutes away. So, although the tide has been rising (not good for clamming), I decided to check it out during the window of time that I had.

Ty and I drove to the Navesink River clam spot and when we got there it was already under water. No good. We decided to take a look at another area open for clamming on the Shrewsbury River that was only a five minute drive away. The tide was about an hour behind our last spot but rising quickly. We would only have about 30 minutes to find some clams. I went into the water with my waders about knee deep and literally within one minute I found my first clam - a big, hard shell cherry-stone (or quahog). Success!

It seems that we found another good spot because I found about a dozen similar clams in about 20 minutes. As we were preparing to leave to go pick up Jamie, I noticed several small holes in the sand at the waterline. I dug into the sand in back of a hole and as I lifted, a spurt of water came shooting up. Steamers! Ty and I hit the clam jackpot. We spent another five to ten minutes digging around all of these small holes and in that short period of time we found about two dozen steamers. I was very excited and Ty had a blast (literally, he got blasted in the face with a shot of water from a clam). These clams would be enough to hold me over until Thursday or Friday when I could find some time to go out and try again for some fish.

That's about it for Day 1. A lot of success - clams for a week, plenty of salt, rice and bean rations. I'm on my way. I'll get into the greens on Day 2.

Day 2 - The Headache

"Stay away from people who belittle your ambition. Small people always do that. The really great people make you feel like you too can be great."
~Mark Twain

Uuuugggh - What a day. Debbie told me to expect this but did I listen? Nope. I woke up with a mild headache today that progressively got worse and worse and worse and worse (how many times can I write worse?) and worse throughout the day and when I got home from work it was still there.

After dinner, still there. At about 8:30 pm I laid down to watch TV and I fell asleep within a half hour. Magically, it went away in my sleep. Thank god.

Why? Well, apparently this is part of the "detox" process.

Day 2 was my first long day at work (8am - 7pm) and I have to admit it was a rough one. I'm almost thankful for work because it allowed me to take my mind off my hunger and my headache for brief times throughout the day. I was so excited about the successes of Day 1 that I wasn't fully prepared for this little wall that I hit on Day 2. Already??? It's only been two days and I feel so hungry and my energy was drained and my head was pounding!

Last night for dinner I cooked a cup of rice and a cup of beans and luckily I had enough of that left to make a lunch for myself at work. In the morning before work I quickly steamed one of my large clams, trimmed it up a bit and mixed it into my rice and beans lunch. And yeah - you know I put my special sea salt on top. Before I got into my truck to go to work I pulled up a patch of wild garlic and a few dandelion greens from the backyard, threw them into my lunch and I was on my way. I just needed to add a few greens to my lunch. It was small. All day at work I was thinking about food.

When I got home I had a variety of "lawn greens" as part of my dinner, accompanied by - you guessed it - beans and rice and clams, clams, clams. This batch was half of my remaining steamers so I still have more for tomorrow. Steamers just aren't the same without the drawn butter! The salt helps a lot though. I will be looking forward to butter as a reward next week. I grossed the kids out a little when I started dissecting the clam bellies at the table. I still have a hard time eating some parts of these clams. The bellies have this mushy center and a dark part that the kids are convinced is clam poop. And I pulled out this clear worm-like organ from each one and wiggled it in front of them before slurping it like a piece of spaghetti (no taste to that part).

With Debbie's help I learned about a variety of common lawn weeds that are especially nutritious and edible. I already knew a lot about dandelions but here's something very interesting - I learned today that you will have a hard time finding a more nutritious green: dandelion leaves have more calcium and iron than spinach, more beta-carotene than carrots, and are loaded with other vitamins and minerals as well.

Also growing in my yard are Blue Violet (Viola papilionacea), Plantain (Plantago major – not plantain bananas) and some type of wild mustard garlic weed. Apparently these are all edible. I washed some off and gingerly tasted each one. The Blue Violet was a pretty purple flower and was not bad at all. The leaves were a little bitter. These plants take a bit of getting used to and without salad dressing or seasoning it is not easy. But ya do what ya gotta do to survive.

I should make a point to note here that my lawn is not treated with pesticides. Be careful where you decide to forage for your plant foods. Make sure that there are no chemicals used to treat the plant life in your gathering zones. If you are unsure, just don't risk it. Most well-manicured lawns are probably loaded with chemicals. If it looks too clean - stay away.

DAY 3 – SASHIMI

Waking up today without a headache was the best start I could have asked for. Anyone who has suffered from headaches knows exactly what I'm talking about.

Breakfast today – well, I was out of cooked rice and beans and I didn't feel like having clams for breakfast so I just picked on some of the leftover greens from yesterday. It wasn't much but I usually don't eat much for breakfast anyway. Today is Wednesday and once a week I have allowed myself a sashimi lunch as part of the rules of my challenge. Let me explain why. . .

(This may sound like a cop out but hey - I made the rules so I don't really care).

Because I have to work during the week (and long hours on Tuesday and Wednesday) I don't have the time to get outside midweek to gather stuff to eat. I sometimes don't even have time to prepare meals in advance but it is even harder when I have to find the meals. So I gave myself this one "out" each week for lunch in the middle of the work week. If I didn't, I would be totally drained of energy at work and I just can't let that happen. So there you have it. I chose sashimi because it's the closest thing to eating what I normally would eat in this diet anyway. Plus, it's the healthiest meal ever, I love it and it gives me something to mentally look forward to.

Lunch - sashimi (2 pieces each of tuna, white tuna, yellowtail, salmon, and mackerel), a small salad, small bowl of brown rice, green tea, and I used a little soy and wasabi.

Dinner - Well, it's back to clams. I had half a pot of steamers left so I cooked them. I took three of them out before cooking because I wanted to see how they tasted raw. A steamer clam is actually a miniature version of the giant clam - or geoduck. I love to order this in sushi bars when available so I decided to make a mini-sashimi dish out of the raw necks of these clams. They turned out pretty good. I was a little worried about pollution in the Shrewsbury River but I have to trust the areas that are marked by the state as safe water for clamming. Last week I did some telephone research with the department of health and the water/shellfish board, and they explained how and where they check the NJ waters. It made me feel more comfortable taking clams from these waters.

I used the cooked clams along with some broth, sea salt and a couple pieces of wild garlic greens to make a small bowl of clam soup. It was good. I will need to cook some more rice and beans for tomorrow.

Day 4 – Clamming

"Unless you try something beyond what you have already mastered, you will never grow."

~ Ronald E. Osborn

I headed out this evening to restock my clam supply. Went with Ty, and friends Pat and Jonah and we hit the end of low tide so there wasn't too much sand left to dig for steamers. Surprisingly we did quite well. This spot is very good. I stocked up on some big cherrystones and a bunch of steamers and also collected some large worms to use for bait tomorrow. Foul weather is coming so I have to try to get out early to see if I can put a fish in my belly for the weekend. That would be a huge help.

With all of these clams, I'm really missing butter! There's only so much you can do with them without any seasonings other than salt. I broiled some clam strips last night for dinner - mixed with some rice and beans. A little butter and pepper would have gone really well with that. If I haven't said it enough already, I'm looking forward to my reward on Monday.

Creatively cooking the same things in different ways is an interesting learning experience.

Day 4 – Catching Up and Falling Behind

I finally caught up on my log to document my experiences. Some days it is difficult to live life (taking care of family, work, home, etc.), do my Survivor Diet Challenge (finding food, cooking, eating, storing, planning) and document the whole process. A few days have gone by and I'm catching up – trying to remember what I did and what I ate. I'll try to be more consistent so that the details are not lost.

Today I had to get up at 5 am for work. I guess I'll be skipping the photo session on Thursdays. And breakfast too for that matter.

I put some brown rice that I cooked last night into a container to take to work. I left a little bag of sea salt at work so I can use that for seasoning. I have been periodically snacking on some rice here and there. Not feeling overwhelmingly hungry though - that's good.

The initial weather report for this weekend is not looking too optimistic for fishing. Not good. Somehow or another I need to get out on the water and at least give it a try.

Day 5 - Gone Fishing

"Failure is the opportunity to begin again more intelligently - keep moving forward."

~ Henry Ford

I woke up this morning with high hopes of catching some type of fish for the grill. The weather was threatening to rain all morning but I decided to throw caution to the wind and take the boat out. I grabbed a handful of beans from the fridge for breakfast and brought some clams and worms with me for bait. Today was the first day out on the boat this season so that in itself is usually an adventure. Something always goes wrong with either the engine or the steering or the trailer or one of the other hundred things that could go wrong on a boat. What was it going to be this year?

I neglected to winterize my engine and I didn't even take the batteries out for winter storage or charging. However, despite my lack of winter care, the engine started right up and never had a problem. Amazing! Everything ran perfectly - but there were no fish!

It was really windy and choppy so there was no chance at all of going out to the ocean. I stayed in the main channel of the Shrewsbury River and tried catching a striped bass by drifting with worms on one rod and clams on another. Nothing - not even a nibble. I briefly tried jigging for bass or blues to no avail. I used some of my time on the water to test out my new live well set up and it worked. Not great - but pretty good.

When I got home I was frustrated and hungry so I immediately headed back out to try to find a local trout stream. It is called Hotchhochkins Brook and is about 15 minutes away. I found a couple decent access points where I could park the truck and walk to the stream. I was there for about 2 hours. Not a single nibble. I totally SUCK at fishing. The newspaper today had pictures of kids of all ages holding all of these big trout. Me? Nothing! So in the past week or two I've gone flounder fishing twice, trout fishing three times, striper fishing once and have not had a single bite! Not a bite. That's frustrating. I'm either going to all the wrong places, going at the wrong times, or I just don't know what the hell I'm doing. I think it's probably a combination of all three - and not knowing what the hell I'm doing is very frustrating when I'm trying to get something done.

At least I found a clam spot. Clams. I'm totally starting to get sick of them. I have run out of ways to prepare clams using just salt. I tried mixing a little maple syrup in with some clam strips to see if that would taste any good. I made the maple syrup by draining sap from our maple tree in the back yard in March and then boiling the sap down until all that was left was syrup - almost exactly how I got the salt from the ocean water.

Sap will only run from maple trees toward the end of winter. From what I learned, it's best to collect sap when the temperature drops below freezing at night but raises above freezing during the day. This past winter I drilled a couple holes in a large maple and filled several buckets full of sap. After boiling down it only yielded a couple pints of syrup but it was a cool experiment and I was happy to have some left over for my challenge.

The syrup clams were different. Not good, but not terrible either. I don't really know what I was expecting. It still tasted like clams. I think I would really enjoy fried clams with cocktail sauce or clam cakes or clam chowder! Yummmmm. But all the extra ingredients for those things are not available to me.

I have been demoted to mere "gatherer" status today; the hunter – unsuccessful.

I am feeling a bit stuck right now. The weekend weather looks crappy and even if it was nice out, I don't know where, when, or how to catch a fish anyway. I've got to keep trying. I've gone through about 2 cups each of beans and rice so far. That ration seems to be a good pace. We'll see.

DAY 6 - FISH? HARDLY.

"To get what we've never had before, we must do what we have never done before."

~ Unknown

What can I say about Day 6? It's Saturday. Ty had his first baseball game at 8:30 in the morning and the weather was threatening rain but it never did happen. It was a cold and dreary morning and the ocean and river were basically out of the question for fishing. I still had a nice supply of clams but that's not going to sustain me for much longer. Plus I'm getting sick of them.

I had a little bowl of beans for breakfast and I picked a few more edibles from the lawn as well. I watched 'Survivorman' on TV yesterday and he was showing how grass can be used for nutrition. Instead of eating it, he just picked a wad of grass and chewed it up and sucked out the juices (almost like chewing tobacco). He said the chlorophyll was great for you. So I did that a little in my yard. It wasn't bad - until it came time to spit it out. I had tiny bits of grass stuck between my teeth and it was a little annoying. I suppose it's worth it for the nutritious value though.

I found a nice cluster of freshly sprouting dandelions in the side yard. They are most tender and least bitter at this stage. That was my mid-afternoon snack - sprinkled with a little salt.

Since the saltwater fishing was out, I decided to give the trout another try. Ty wanted to come this time so we headed over to a little pond about 10 minutes away. I chopped up some clam pieces to use for bait. After a while without a bite we switched spots to see if there were any sunfish or other panfish around. They are usually pretty easy to catch. I casted out to a promising spot and sure enough I got a bite. I reeled it in and it was a small catfish. I don't particularly like catfish but beggars can't be choosers. I didn't have a bucket or a bag to put it in so I just put it into my jacket pocket. Ty was pretty excited about that. We continued this way for a while and caught a few tiny sunfish. Into the pocket they all went. I felt a little ridiculous keeping these tiny fish but that's what surviving is all about.

When we got home I dumped out my pocket and all the fish were dead except for the little catfish. They are tough little buggers. The kids were amazed that it had survived for about an hour in my pocket no worse for wear. They begged me not to kill it because they wanted it now for a pet. I caved in (despite my hunger) and we made a little fish bowl setup for this catfish who was promptly named, "Mr. Fredrickson" by Ty. The strange name stuck and the kids have a new pet.

The sunfish were scaled and cleaned and sautéed up with a little salt (man I need some butter or oil). I mixed in some clam pieces and some beans and clam broth. It wasn't bad. If I was REALLY hungry I suppose I would have picked at the bones a little more but I just didn't have the stomach for it. You need butter to really crisp up the fins so that didn't happen either. I was just thankful to have a little fish added to my diet. I think I'll try another lake tomorrow morning. A nice trout would go a long way.

If the weather looks better tomorrow I may go take a look at the ocean or that other lake. What else can I do? Maybe I need to start expanding my search for food. I've focused so much on fish because last year it was quite plentiful but this year I'm having problems. Debbie was reading about some other wild edibles that grow in the salt marsh so maybe I'll give that a try tomorrow.

DAY 7 - ONE WEEK DOWN!

"Do not live in fear of what the future may hold. Live in the anticipation of the new opportunities that lie ahead."
                                        ~ Unknown

I woke up this morning and went right out to Takanassee Lake because I thought there may be a chance to catch a trout for lunch. Ha! Boy was I mistaken. I counted a hundred casts with my little gold spinner before I left (freezing my ass off). Should I just give up my quest for trout?

On my way home I drove past the beach to check the water conditions. It was really rough in shore but the west wind today should calm things down later in the day and maybe tomorrow. I saw a huge fleet of boats about five miles off the beach - presumably fishing for stripers because the reports of great striper fishing have been continuous. I'm not even going to check the reports today because I'm sick of hearing about how thousands of other people are catching fish and I can't get out there.

I'm going tomorrow - out to sea. Going with dad and we're optimistic. I do get quite sea sick on long ocean voyages and this one may be a long one. I feel comfortable that the boat will run well after my initial trip the other day. You never know though.

Ok, so I didn't have much to eat today. I finished my cooked beans and I have to soak the next batch for 4 hours before I can cook them for another hour and a half. (Beans are a tedious project) I'm trying to be careful because the bean container seems to be dwindling quickly. I picked a few greens but not much. Wow - I really didn't have much at all today. I thought I would feel hungrier but I'm not. I'm only hungry when I see food on TV or all the wasted food that my kids don't finish. That's another story.

Guess what Ty and I did this evening? You guessed it - we went clamming again. We hit the tide just right and were quite successful again with both hard cherrystones and steamers. I saw a few crabs when I was there. They were small but this may be an area to check out in the summertime. It was a beautiful night (a little chilly) and it looked amazing when the sun was setting. I tried to take some pictures but they didn't turn out as nice as it really was.

For now I am still stuck with clams. But at least there are clams because without them I would be in trouble. Clam season ends April 30th so I need to get my act together by then.

Tomorrow I have reason to celebrate - one week is done. My reward for surviving one week is a pound of butter and some other spices. The taste will be back in my food. Thank god! I really think this will help a lot but I have to be careful - that butter has to last a long time.

And tomorrow is going to bring fish - a big one. One that will last a long time.

DAY 8 - THE DAY OF THE STRIPED BASS

"Whatever the mind can believe and conceive, it can achieve."
~ Napoleon Hill

I got a good night's sleep - looking forward to my upcoming fishing adventure with dad. Woke up and had some clams for breakfast. No, not your ordinary clams - these had butter, salt and pepper!!! What a difference. The photo I took looked like a pan full of worms but it's just the steamer clam necks sautéed in some butter. Did I mention how happy I am about the butter yet? I think I deserve it after a week of bland chewy clams.

I also had something else interesting today: pine needle tea. Ty picked me a bunch of pine needles from a tree and I just brewed them in a pot of water for a while, strained the needles and had some tea. Supposedly this is very good for you. Not the best tasting tea in the world - but not the worst either. How about that for breakfast? Pine needle tea and sautéed clam strips.

So, I bet you want to know why this is "The Day of the Striped Bass" huh? Well - remember all of the previous talk about how I suck at fishing, yadda yadda yadda. Not today!

I went out with dad and we certainly had an adventure. It started out very questionable though. Should we go? It's windy, should we stay? Where should we go? What are we gonna do? Etc. We bundled up expecting some foul wind and weather - we were very prepared. Luckily, the weather threw us a pleasant curve ball. The wind came from the west and ocean currents were with us. We had about a 25 mile ride ahead and in a small boat you have to really pick your days wisely.

Well, it took some time to get to our spot. In reality this is about two miles right off the beach near my home. But to get there by boat you have to travel 12 miles north, around Sandy Hook, then 12 miles south. It's a pain in the ass, and I hardly ever make the trip because I hate the ride to get there. I am going to find a way to get my kayak to the beach so I can do a two mile paddle rather than a 25 mile boat ride.

Ok, so we located a few party boats and figured we would travel close to them to try to see if anyone was catching. We saw a few fish readings on my sonar but nothing overly impressive. Then we started to see several boats all around us start to hook up with fish and we thought it was about to turn on. Dad had one on for about a minute but then it came loose. Crap! Then, all of a sudden they were gone. I didn't have a bite at all. We were using metal jigs because the reports said they were catching most of the fish that way.

We hit a lull and it lasted for a couple of hours. All of the other boats left. We were alone out there and it was getting late. We talked about going home but I NEEDED to catch at least one striper. We continued just driving around searching for some sign of life by looking at the sonar/fish-finder. Our moods were very low and we were so close to giving up. Then, all of a sudden we started seeing some marks on the fish-finder. This is what we were waiting and searching and hoping for all day!

We started dropping our jigs down again and suddenly, it was ON! It was one of the most exciting displays of fishing you would ever want to be part of. We were sitting smack dab in the middle of a school of feeding striped bass that were all about 20 pounds. They were chasing anything we threw at them and within five minutes we boated our four fish limit. Then it was just fishing for fun. One after the other, 20+ pound stripers! It was truly amazing and exciting and it was a fantastic experience to share with my dad.

We've had a lot of unlucky fishing trips and this one started to look like we would add another skunk to the list. But it all turned around and we were in striped bass central for about a half hour. Great time - I'm so glad we persevered and kept searching and searching.

I never thought I would be throwing back 20 pound fish during my Survivor Diet Challenge but the limit is two per man so we kept our first four and must have released another six during this frenzy. Dad took one home, I'm planning on giving one of them to my friendly neighborhood sushi chef (to see if he'll hook me up with some free sushi in exchange), and the other two will be filleted tomorrow night after sitting on ice for a day. It's tempting to cut right into one for dinner but I know from experience that the meat is much better if it's chilled for 24 hours on ice. So it's clams and rice and beans for another night. But just knowing I have a bounty of striped bass in waiting gives me a significant mental boost.

That brings up a good point about my situation. A good part of this challenge is the mental game. When you are struggling to find food you are constantly thinking of new things to try. This keeps the mind active. Normally, on lazy weekend day I would check the fridge for a snack and then veg out on the couch in front of the television and most likely take a nap. Bad news. When you're in survivor mode there is absolutely no time for that whatsoever.

On the flip side, when you're struggling your mind does get a little depressed. Not knowing where or when the next meal will be is a humbling experience to say the least. These are the times that separate the survivors from the rest of the pack. Survivors persevere. Adapt.

Knowing that I have fish for the next few days takes off a tremendous amount of mental pressure. I feel like I can go about my regular life for a while in a normal capacity. I have to remember not to get too comfortable though. After all, it's only Day 8 and there's still a long road ahead.

Day 9 - Farewell Mr. Fredrickson

"Tis not the meat but the appetite that makes eating a delight."
~ Sir John Suckling

It will be a long day ahead at work. It was easier knowing that I had some nice striped bass in the cooler on ice - ready to fillet when I got home. That wasn't going to be until 7:30 pm. And I had about an hour of cleaning to do before I could even start cooking. I had my regular beans and rice for lunch at work.

At lunchtime I took a ride over to my regular sushi restaurant and I gave them one of the big striped bass that I had on ice. I didn't stay but I am hopeful that my generosity will be reciprocated the next time I go there - maybe they will trade a nice fillet of yellowtail to me in exchange. I'm not expecting anything, but we'll see. In the past I've sold striped bass to restaurants (when I lived in RI) and I could get about $60 per fish.

The kids were excited to tell me all about how they let Mr. Fredrickson go back home. Apparently they got tired of cleaning the fish tank (or cake pan in this case) and Debbie brought them all to the pond where he was from. Farewell Mr. Fredrickson.

After work I went home and got to work . . . on the fish that is. I was very careful to fillet these fish properly in order to get everything I could from them. After all, they sacrificed their lives for me. It wouldn't be right to do a half-assed cleaning job. This took some time. I prepared the fish for several cooking methods. I made several chunks for the grill (leaving the skin on), several pieces to sauté, a few rib and belly sections for the grill, and a batch of strips that I am going to put on the smoker this weekend. I got a good amount of meat from these two fish and I will do my best to make it last because there's no telling when the next fish will be available. After I was finished cleaning I had to go down to the river to dump the guts and bones. In hindsight I should have kept some bone pieces to make a fish stock. Dummy! I'll remember that for next time.

I vacuum bagged several portions of fish and froze some to keep it as fresh as possible. For dinner tonight I seasoned two rib sections and a belly section with salt and pepper and spread some melted butter on it. I put the pieces on a hot grill and they turned out excellent! Ty has been thoroughly enjoying eating my meals with me lately. He dug right in to this fish. The skin was nice and crispy and flavorful and the flesh was juicy, tender, large, white meat flakes. So good. For those who don't know, the rib and belly sections are commonly discarded by most fishermen who catch and fillet their own fish. It's a disgrace because this meat has so much flavor. It's just a little more inconvenient to prepare but if you have the time, it's worth it - especially on these larger fish.

Well, that's it for tonight. I have plenty of fish for a few days. I still have a bunch of clams in the fridge – I'll have to cook those tomorrow. I think I really have to concentrate my efforts on the greens next. I have definitely been lacking in that department.

DAY 10 - SURVIVING THE DAY AT WORK

"The quality of an individual is reflected in the standards they set for themselves."

~ Ray Kroc

I had to rush a bit this morning because I had a long day ahead. I work until 6:00 and then I have a digital photography class after work. I had to get my camera together, make lunch, steam some clams, vacuum pack some more fish fillets and get ready for work. I was in a rush and left the kitchen a whirlwind - sorry Deb, I'll clean up later. I got to work and at some point in the mid-morning a delivery box arrived and was sitting on our lunch table. It had a Dr Cuozzo label on it so it must have been from his office. I opened it up and inside were the biggest, most delicious looking, plump, red, juicy strawberries dipped in deep dark chocolate! All the salivary glands under my tongue kicked into overdrive. I had a hard time containing my public display of salivation. They said Dr Cuozzo's mom made them but I don't know - this looked like a professional job!

Anyone who knows me also knows that the chocolate covered strawberry is one of my top, if not THE top food weakness for me. Even when I'm not on a food restrictive diet I have a hard time stopping myself from eating every last one of them when they are around. I just had to sit there and watch all of the women in the office enjoying the chocolaty goodness. One of them bit into a berry and a big hunk of chocolate fell off and onto the floor! I know she wanted to call a "ten second rule" but she thought better and tossed it in the garbage. Tossed it in the garbage! Tossed it in the garbage. Tossed it in the garbage. Tossed it in the garbage. Tossed it in the garbage. Whoops. Sorry, I guess my mind was somewhere else.

Then, later in the day a patient came in and brought a container of fresh hummus and crackers for the staff as a gift. So very generous. I shouldn't be rude. Right? I mean, it would be quite insulting of me not to at least taste these gifts so that I can give a proper 'thank you' to the givers.

Well, I have to tell you - the road of temptation is a dangerous one to follow. First it's a little cracker with hummus - then a chocolate covered strawberry - then another and another. Where does it end??? Admittedly,

I have had a couple minor "cheats and steals" along the way. Like a teaspoon of olive oil here, and a small piece of cut up pineapple there. Nobody's perfect. I'm trying to keep a very accurate account of my inappropriate behavior and I am planning to reveal that in an upcoming log entry. (I don't think anyone wants to see that - do you?) However - I made a conscious effort this morning to say, "No more cheats!" and this batch of strawberries has really put my will power to the test.

I don't know. It's all so confusing sometimes. I mean what could be the harm of just grabbing a tiny bite of something I really enjoy from time to time. NO. Stop it - you're trying to get me to cave. Well it's not going to happen. Uh-Oh. Talking to myself now. I think I better get back to work. I'm starting to lose it.

DAY 11 - THE NEED FOR GREEN

"Don't measure yourself by what you haven't accomplished - but by what you plan to accomplish."

~ John Wooden (partial)

I got on the scale this morning and it read 179. Down 11 pounds from my 190 starting point. So that's 11 pounds in 11 days. Interesting. I'm not really intent on losing a bunch of weight with this diet and about 175 is as low as I really want to go. I figure if I go to 175 then after I stop the diet I will probably put back on about 5-10 pretty easily. So my target weight is ideally somewhere between 180-185.

That being said, I am going to have to figure out how to stay on this diet until the end - without losing any more weight (once I hit 175ish). Hmmm. Another challenge. Perhaps I will add a few chocolate covered strawberries to my daily dessert. (See - I just can't let that go from yesterday.) I might have to add something - it should be healthy. It should be something survivorish. And it should help keep the weight on. I need some ideas.

Remember I mentioned a few cheats that I have had since I started? I do feel a little guilty about that. It really wasn't much - just a few little bites of things here and there. Well, in exchange, I gave up my sushi lunch luxury reward this week. I REALLY look forward to that too. And I haven't seen my sushi guy since I gave him that big fish. I'll go back there next week. I hope that eases my guilt a bit from my bad behavior - that's my penance.

For breakfast/lunch today I cooked up a little fish before work. I was up cooking fish fillets at 5:45 in the morning. I figured out a great way to quickly cook some bass pieces that come out so tender and delicious. After cleaning all the fish, I made several sections that I can use like rations. I had a piece this morning that I cut up into little 'nuggets,' for lack of a better word. I did this before I cooked them, heated some butter in a pan, seasoned with sea salt and pepper and then seared each nugget on each side. It was similar to how I cook scallops - getting that nice caramelized crust on the outside yet moist and tender on the inside. It's fast and it's delicious. Of course Ty loves it too so I'm lucky to get half of what I cook when he's lurking about. I brought some of my fish nuggets to work and I picked on them throughout the day.

I think I'm done with steamers for a while. I bit into one yesterday that had this hard, grittiness inside one piece. Not only did I fear breaking a tooth but it just turned me off from them altogether for a while. I still have some larger cherrystones in the fridge and I'm sure they will be fine for another couple days. There is only about one more week left for clamming season before it is illegal so I'll probably get back out there once more to stock up on some of the cherrystones if I can.

Protein, protein, protein. That's all I've been eating lately. I need some more diversity and I need some more green veggies. Later today I am going to do some foraging and pick myself a big salad. I'll have a fish salad for dinner. Sounds good.

DAY 11 - BLUES IN THE BACKYARD

"Never leave fish."

~ Gary Peterson

I had to add another post to Day 11 because of this very exciting event (if you're a fisherman). This is basically a long fishing report.

After work I took Jamie out in the kayak. At the end of my street there is a beach access to the Branchport Creek of the Shrewsbury River. I rigged a bicycle-kayak trailer so I can get some exercise when I go kayak fishing. Anyway, we put the kayak in the water, basically in my backyard and as we started paddling out we saw the splashes of many fish all around.

I could tell these were bunker schools by the sounds they were making when they were breaking water. This is a little early in the season for bunker but it has been early for everything so far. They were EVERYWHERE! I had two rods with me and luckily I brought some treble hooks for snagging.

Jamie was casting shad jigs while I was rigging the other rod with a treble. She's a great caster for a 7 year old girl. However, at one point the reel seat came loose and as she went to cast I glanced over and the reel went flying into the river! She was holding the rod and the bail was still open on the reel which was at the bottom of the river. I've never seen that happen in my life. In order to retrieve this reel we had to paddle FAR away as ALL the line came off the reel. I knew I tied a knot on the spool. When we got to the end I had to hand pull up all of the line - dragging a seaweed covered reel to the kayak. Picture me and Jamie sitting in the kayak, covered with 6 lb test fishing line, trying desperately to feed all the line into the water so that it doesn't get tangled up. Eventually it got tangled. I did retrieve the reel, cut the tangled mess, retied and salvaged as much line as I could. Whoooh! Then after all that Jamie looks at me and says, "I want to go home - I'm cold."

Ok - so you may be wondering why I went into so much detail there. Well, the whole time this reel/line fiasco thing is going on, there are bunker splashing ALL AROUND ME! And every couple minutes there was a major attack from big predator fish. I did everything I could to contain myself and help to fix this reel/real problem.

Not that I don't love when my kids come fishing with me, but I was very happy to paddle back to drop Jamie off so that I could get back to serious business! I re-rigged both rods for live bait fishing and I was ready. The tide was the highest I've ever seen it in this area. It was about 5:00 pm and I stayed out there until 9:00. It was non-stop as these massive schools of bunker attracted the big bluefish. There may have been bass there too but I only saw signs of bluefish.

I had a fantastic time. I had multiple tackle foul-ups but that only adds to the excitement when you're in the fish like that. I had a very lightweight trout rod with 6 pound test mono, and I had a medium action spinning rod loaded with 50 lb braid. I figured that would be my main rod but I rigged up both anyway. I didn't use the weighted treble because I didn't have very good leverage from the kayak for snagging fish and my rods weren't heavy enough. Initially I used an 80lb leader tied straight to the big treble hook. After snagging a bunker I repositioned the treble and just let him swim back out. I did manage to snag with the lightweight rod too - there were so many bunker it was crazy. At times I had two live line rods out with a swimming bunker on each. Can you imagine any tackle mishaps at this point - from a kayak?

Both baits got attacked at the same time. I grabbed the larger rod and let him take it for a few seconds. When I went to set the hook, SNAP, my rod broke in half. Not only did the rod break but the line broke as well. So I lost my rod top, my rig and my fish! The bottom of the rod had one guide left. I switched back to the other rod which was bent over and started to reel it in. I couldn't set the hook because of the light rod and as I brought it near, the fish came loose. I reeled it up and the 80 pound mono was cut clean through. Treble hook #2 gone. 2 left. Now I had a half-rod and a lightweight trout rod trying to catch fish that were probably over 10 pounds, using bait fish that were alive and over 10 inches each.

I scrambled through my tackle pouch and luckily found a six-inch wire leader! Yeah - that was going to be a big help. I couldn't cast the half rod so I rigged it with the wire leader and big hook. I retied a treble to the small rod and was on the hunt for bunker again. I had a very tough time because of the flimsy rod but I was eventually able to snag one. I switched it over to the shorty rod and let the bunker swim out. As it was waiting to be eaten, I continued to try to snag with the light rod.

This is probably my favorite kind of fishing. It's so exciting. I watched that bait swim out and I just knew that any minute it was going to be under attack. The bunker started to freak out and that meant something was lurking below. I grabbed the half rod and got ready. Down it went and there was a lot of splashing and thrashing as my bait was fleeing for its life. I gave it a couple seconds and then set the hook. Did you ever try to set the hook from a kayak with only half a rod? Needless to say I didn't exert too much force. I pulled and reeled and what was heavy for a second or two suddenly became loose. I reeled up and on the end of my hook was a bunker head. The blues love to eat bunker tails. Bass eat them headfirst. That's another story.

So now I'm back to square one. Find some bait, snag one, put it out there to be attacked. This time I made a modification to my rig. Attached to my big hook I tied a thick leader with a stinger hook about five inches away. I rigged the bunker with the large hook in its back and then put the small stinger hook in the tail. Almost immediately it was attacked. There was splashing and thrashing and I could see my bait escape the first wave. It was right on top and doing everything it could to escape. And somehow it did! I let it sit out there for a good five minutes longer just bleeding and barely moving. How perfect could that be? Well, while I waited I was able to snag another bunker with the light rod. This was a nice fresh one - very lively. I reeled in my battered bait - he was mauled, slashed and cut but still alive. I took him off the hook, tossed him back and rigged the fresh bait in the same way with the stinger hook.

It was getting dark now and although it had been non-stop action for several hours, these bluefish were beating me. I hadn't landed a single fish and my rod was all broken up and I was freezing. Oh, I forgot to mention that at about 7:00 pm it started down-pouring on me. The rain lasted about 20 minutes so I was thoroughly drenched. My dad's 'life credo' of "Never Leave Fish" went through my mind several times when I thought about quitting. No way was I leaving without a fish!

Well - this latest bait was doing its thing when the attack happened again. Bam, splash, slash - but this time it was really splashing. The fish was hooked! I didn't even have to do anything but reel it in. My stinger hook worked. It's not easy bringing in a 10 pound bluefish with a half rod - in a kayak. I got it to the net after being towed around for a short while and the battle was over. It was dark, I was wet and chilled to the bone, I had my fish - time to go. Very exciting - all in my backyard.

If it had not been for the Survivor Diet Challenge I would have left this area after my first sign of adversity. Well, maybe not the first - but the point is that having the challenge in the back of my mind kept me going. It kept me engaged and kept me thinking and re-inventing new ways to try to accomplish my task.

I don't particularly like bluefish to eat - but I am very proud of myself for what I went through to catch this one. And I am going to eat it and enjoy it and remember what it took to make it all happen. This bluefish will taste better than any other because of the effort.

Day 12 - Smoking Some Fish

"The difficulties and struggles of today are the price we pay for the successes of tomorrow."

~ William J. H. Boetcker

I have a nice batch of striped bass pieces drying in the refrigerator today. Last night I made some brine with water, salt and some maple syrup (almost all gone). I soaked the fish overnight and this morning I laid it all out on a drying rack and put it in the fridge. I am trying to get a pellicle to form. A pellicle is a sticky glaze on the outside of the meat. This will let the smoke adhere to it.

I also have that bluefish on ice and that will go into the smoker/grill probably tomorrow. The brine is just a highly concentrated salt water mixture with some syrup added for flavor and I think I can preserve it to be used over and over again. I keep it in the fridge in a zip top bag and I'll use it again for the bluefish. I won't use it too many times but there's no sense in wasting it if I don't have to.

After work today I'm going to start the smoker up which is basically my gas grill which has been modified a bit. I think I have some apple wood chips in the garage from last year.

For lunch today (and breakfast for that matter) I had a big bowl of sautéed dandelion greens and some beans. Debbie really helped a lot with the greens but was careful to stay within the guidelines.

At first it tasted like a cross between broccoli rabe and spinach. I didn't mind eating it but towards the end the bitter flavor started to repulse me a little.

I actually couldn't finish the last bite and I felt like I did when I was a kid sneaking my unwanted food into a napkin to throw it in the garbage. I love most vegetables but I am fearful that I am going to get awfully tired of these dandelions and wild yard greens. My fig tree plant has sprouted its first cute little figlet. At this rate I will have a handful of figs by Christmas. Oh well. I forced myself to eat a bunch of greens today and hopefully that will sustain me for a while.

I really, really, really want a chocolate bar. And not your ordinary Hershey's bar. I'm thinking of a big block of Valrhona chocolate from Whole Foods. They are so thick that you can't easily open your mouth wide enough to bite a chunk off. It's dark, rich 60-70% chocolate. . . Ok - gotta stop right there. I'm daydreaming/typing again. Sorry to bore you with my thoughts. These aren't the rambling of a starving person but more like the thoughts of someone craving a forbidden fruit. I certainly don't feel like I'm starving. It's just that I miss that taste of chocolate right now and it's not going away.

After work, I went right to 'work' on my smoker and bass strips. I used my gas grill and made an aluminum foil pouch to hold the apple wood chips. I had some trouble getting it to really smoke though. It seemed like it took forever to start the chips smoking and once they did, it wasn't a tremendous amount. Perhaps I need to learn a little more about Apple wood or some of the other types of wood that people use to smoke food. Maybe some woods that are either softer or harder will lend themselves better for getting a good smoke on. I am just a beginner at this but at least I'm trying and even if I fail, that will be an opportunity to begin again but more intelligently the next time around.

It still seemed to work pretty well. My fish strips turned out very good. If I had one criticism it would be that the smoked bass was a little on the salty side. (That sea salt really packs a punch) So when I do the bluefish tomorrow I will rinse off the strips well before I lay them on the rack to dry. See - learning from mistakes.

We had a 'dinner and drinks' get together to attend tonight and although everyone there knew I was doing the SDC it was uncomfortable for me to be in a social setting and not participate in the food and drink. I must have had a gallon of water. I was tempted to put the challenge aside for the night (especially for a beer!) but I think I did the right thing by staying strong. It's actually helpful when everyone knows I'm doing it because they become more supportive. And it's always an interesting topic of conversation - that's for certain.

Two people who have thriving gardens, even this early in the season, invited me over to pick some greens. I think I may take them up on their offers. I don't think that would contradict my rule system - although it's a slight bending of the rules. I was also thinking about the fish that I gave to my sushi place. If I catch fish and then sell or trade them for other food or goods, that is surviving as well. I should be able to use anything that I find, forage, or fish to trade like currency for other things - as long as the other things aren't like a Big Mac and fries. But I think if I trade a striped bass for a fillet of salmon or yellowtail - that would be fine. It would be nice just to have a little more variety and diversity in my diet. Man, I could really go for a Guinness right about now!

I am craving comfort foods. I'm glad I didn't ask if they had any Guinness in the fridge because if they said yes then I may have jumped ship. All in all I think I did very well being out in a social setting with food and drink abound. Will-power and supportive friends will go a long way during this challenge.

DAY 13 - MASTERING THE SMOKER

"It's the amount that you do over and beyond what's required of you that determines your degree of success."

~ *Unknown*

Although it is Saturday there is no rest for the weary. It is kids' baseball day! Ty has a game at 8:30 am followed by Jamie's at 11. Debbie is doing some work this morning so I am on baseball duty.

It was fun but we were rushed in the morning which made it difficult for me to eat breakfast. I quickly sautéed some striped bass pieces - quite delicious. I'm getting pretty good at that and the way I slice it makes it cook very quickly.

I grabbed a bottle of water and we were off for the whole morning. After Ty's game we went to Jersey Mike's Subs to get the kids some lunch to go. This was very difficult for me because I REALLY wanted a sub. They make pretty classic subs there with seasonings and oil and vinegar which soaks into the bread just perfectly. I watched the kids eat them and watched lettuce and tomatoes fall out on the ground as they were biting. Uhg! I really wanted a big bite of that sub.

After the games I was getting pretty hungry. When we got home I did another bass sauté the same way as breakfast and put on a pot of rice. I think I'm doing ok with my rations so far and I should be eating more rice than I have been lately. The smoked bass strips were all gone because I munched on them all night last night while watching television. I've heard that it's not very good for you to eat too much smoked food because of its carcinogenic potential. I will try to limit that a little more, but I look forward to the upcoming bluefish.

While the rice was cooking I took out the dried bluefish and it had a nice sticky pellicle so I seasoned it with pepper and it was smoking time again.

I didn't like the gas grill after what happened yesterday with the bass so I decided to clean up the Weber charcoal grill and give that a try. I got about 10 coals started up in the chimney. While that was going I soaked a Ziploc bag full of wood chips to get them saturated for the smoker. I also added the charred wood chips that were left over from the gas grill figuring they would add to the process. I made a tin foil pan and filled the bottom with soaked chips and then I put a layer of piping hot coals on top of that and then covered it with another layer of wood chips. I positioned all of the fish strips on the rack and almost immediately the chips started smoking. I covered the grill and let it do its thing for about two hours. The temperature never got above 200 (perfect) and the amount of smoke was insane. Just what I was looking for and what I was lacking with the gas grill.

When the fish was done, Ty and I gave it a taste. It was excellent. Not too salty (after a thorough rinsing beforehand) and still quite tender. Not a hint of fishiness (because I was very careful to cut out all of the red meat in the bluefish) and just the right amount of smoky flavor. That was definitely the way to get the smoker going.

I didn't overdo it on the smoked bluefish. I want that to last for a while so I bagged it up and put it in the fridge. I can snack on that whenever I get the urge. I just have to keep Ty from gobbling it all up. For dinner I had previously defrosted a nice piece of striped bass with the skin on.

My goal was to cook it so that the skin got nice and crispy on the outside. It worked pretty well and it was a fantastic dinner.

I went out to the yard to look for more of those Violet flowers. Not only are those flowers quite sweet and tasty, the greens that come off of them are very good too. They don't have that abrasive bitterness that the dandelion green or that mustard garlic has. It's a very 'lettuce' like flavor. I picked a bunch of those greens and made a bed of them on my plate. I put the bass fillet on top, added some brown rice and a piece of smoked bluefish - and topped it all off with a few of the pretty sweet purple flowers. Now this was a dinner that I could have regularly! I actually think Debbie was a little jealous of my meal compared to hers.

Back to clams again tomorrow - I still have about eight cherrystones in the fridge needing to be cooked. Maybe I'll try something different for breakfast. I have to remember to take out another ration of striped bass from the freezer tomorrow too. Maybe I'll cook that other rib section tomorrow afternoon.

I will have survived two weeks tomorrow. Still going strong but I have been tested several times already. My will power is waning and I need to stay mentally strong at this point in the challenge. My temptation to cheat and steal leftovers from the kids is very strong I must admit. Recently this has become more of a mental challenge than a physical one. Overall I feel pretty good but this afternoon I was feeling a little energy drained while playing ball with Ty. I took a mid-afternoon nap and that seemed to help revitalize me. I just have to stay the course and keep moving forward.

Although the kids are mostly supportive, there are times when they find it funny to be a tease. When they know I can't have something the have a little fun dangling the carrot in front of my face (so to speak). I'll get them back. Maybe not right now but someday soon, I'll get them back.

DAY 14 - I HATE DAY 14

"Whatever the mind can believe and conceive, it can achieve."
~ Napoleon Hill

I don't have a whole lot to do today. It's raining outside so I'm stuck inside and my kids have a recent fascination with the TV Food Network. Granted it's better than Nickelodeon or goofy cartoons but the food, the food, the FOOD! It all looks sooooooo good. Ace of Cakes, Good Eats, The Best Thing I Ever Ate! Come on! All I want is something sweet and savory and my meal plan just ain't cutting it.

I only have about two tablespoons of maple syrup left and that's the only sweet thing I have. The problem is I can't make any more of that because the sap is not running anymore. I even put a little syrup on my rice this morning for breakfast.

Speaking of breakfast, I busted open the last of the clams - they were still perfectly fine after spending about a week in the fridge. I cleaned them and chopped them up and sautéed them with some butter and then added some rice and a crumbled up piece of smoked bluefish. All together it was actually quite good. Not chocolate cake good, but quite good.

Throughout the day I managed to gobble up ALL of my reserve smoked bluefish - just because it was there. It's no cookie but it's the closest thing to sweet that I had. I'm really jonesing for some desserty foods. Well, it's not over yet - maybe I can figure something out. Who says you can't have chocolate cake on the SDC? Maybe not chocolate cake exactly - but something . . . just have to think.

(long pause)

I did some thinking and some research and came up with bupkis! The only sweets from nature that I could come up with were sugar cane - which, to my knowledge, doesn't grow around here, or honey. Honey is a good idea - if I want to risk being stung to death by bees! I don't have any idea where to find a beehive or even if there are bees making honey at this time of year? I suppose that once the flowers start blooming the bees start making. Well, I'm not that desperate yet. But I will certainly bee keeping my eyes open. We'll see.

For dinner I had defrosted two rib sections from one of the striped bass I caught earlier in the week. I had my mind set on grilling them but after I lit the grill I had a disaster! I looked out the window and the front of my grill was on fire! Ty thought it was the coolest thing. I quickly shut off the gas valve at the house and the fire went out. I had caught it in time before it caused any major damage but my gas line is melted and I won't be able to use the gas grill until I fix it.

I moved the fish ribs to the toaster oven and set it to broil. It wasn't quite the same as grilled, but it turned out fine. I ate one and I picked all the meat off the other for tomorrow's breakfast or lunch. I can't believe that most people usually throw away this part of the fish. There's so much meat in this area and it's very good quality meat at that. It just takes some extra care to clean it.

Day 15 - Keeping Busy

"Things turn out the best for the people who make the best of the way things turn out."

~ *John Wooden*

Today I was dreading the fact that I really didn't have much to do and the weather report was once again forecasting rain and yuck. However, I got through it fairly easily by finding some stuff to do around the house that I had been procrastinating about. In the middle of the day there was about a two hour break in the rain and drear so I used that opportunity to hop on the kayak for a little exercise and I was pleasantly surprised at the result.

I trolled two rods out the side of the kayak using plastic storm shad lures and started paddling non-stop. To start, I paddled right into the wind and almost immediately got a bite on one of my rods. It was a big fish! Then as quickly as it was there, it was gone - my line had been cut. Bluefish. It took me a while to get situated again but soon enough I was trolling again. This time I toughened up my tackle by adding 80 pound test to one rod and a wire leader to the other.

It took some time but eventually I got another strike. This time it was on! My tactic of beefing up my tackle seemed to work perfectly and after a good fight with a lot of jumps, I landed a nice sized bluefish. It got all tangled in my other line and I almost booted it while trying to get it into the net - but it all worked out in the end.

I was excited to have these two opportunities because I thought today was going to be a total wash. I immediately started the troll up again but after about an hour of paddling - no more bites. I wanted one more fish so badly because I could have smoked one and had the other as regular meals. I'm not sure what I'll do with this one but the smoker worked so well last time I'm sure I will do some that way. I started getting rained on quite a bit so I packed it in and went home. My home-made kayak trailer for my bicycle works great!

I put the fish in a bag and stuck the whole thing in the refrigerator (sorry Deb) so that it will be ready to fillet tomorrow after work.

Monday is one of my nights to make a family dinner. I decided to make a veggie stir fry with chicken and noodles. Debbie bought some broccoli and bok choy and I cooked up a really wonderful SMELLING dinner. The fresh garlic and ginger and soy sauce have such an aroma. It's always difficult to cook such a meal without eating any. Everyone else seemed to enjoy it though - so that gave me some satisfaction.

For myself I made a fish burger. Sounds great huh? Actually - it was quite delicious. I sautéed up some striped bass and after it cooled I flaked apart the meat and mixed it with a handful of rice. I seasoned with salt and pepper and formed it into a burger-like patty. I browned it in a frying pan with some melted butter and all I was missing was the bun. I think I could have convinced myself that it was actually a burger I was eating - or at least a crab cake. It held together quite well just using the rice and fish.

I regret having Old Bay as one of my weekly rewards from last week because I didn't use it - didn't need it. Salt from the sea and pepper is really all I need for spices. The butter was a blessing. Can you tell by how many times I've mentioned cooking with it? I really have to start rationing the butter because I've gone through one quarter of my supply already in one week having it. At that rate I'll be out of butter before the end of week 5 - so I have to be smart about that. I am going to think about the Old Bay thing. Since I haven't used it, maybe I'll substitute it for something else that I could use. After all - they are my rules and I can change them if I want to.

I almost forgot about my reward for completing week two - flour, bread crumbs and vegetable oil. Hmmm, can you make chocolate chip cookies with that? Ha! Those things should be helpful. I can fry some clams this week if I get anymore. Clam season ends April 30th, so if I want to have a supply I better get out soon. I think Thursday the 29th should be a good low tide after work so I'll make sure to go then.

I got through this day by keeping busy, housework, fishing, kayaking, a lot of cooking, fixing computers, setting up video games for the kids, etc. It's going to be a long day at work tomorrow. Back to beans and rice for lunch.

DAY 16 - WINDBLOWN KAYAK

"Good judgment comes from experience and experience comes from bad judgment."

~ Rita Mae Brown

Breakfast – A glass of water.

Lunch – A bottle of water, container of rice and beans and the smell of a chocolate angel food cake. Mmmmm.

Dinner – A glass of water and a piece of striped bass.

Snacks – Several glasses of water and a handful of beans here and there.

When I got home from work around 7:30 I had the great idea to jump in the kayak for a quick fishing excursion but as I started paddling to my spot the wind picked up quite a bit. I was being pushed sideways so instead of fighting it, I let it take me along as I fished. Little did I think about how I was going to get back home! After about 10 minutes I called it quits - then the real adventure began. I could NOT paddle against this wind. I was going as fast as I could paddle and I was literally going backwards. I was in real trouble here. Luckily I wasn't in any serious danger - just more of an inconvenience. Worst case scenario - I would just get blown across the river until I hit land on the other side. Then I could call Debbie to pick me up in the truck. That was the backup plan. Instead, I paddled on - furiously! I had to hug the river bank to get as much shelter from the wind as I could. That worked for a while but when it came time to cross back over to my side I just kept going backwards. I had to find little breaks in the wind in order to make any progress going across. It took me about an hour to go about 100 yards! Crazy. And every time I got tired and had to rest - yup, you guessed it - I was blown back and my progress was all lost.

My kayak totally sucks in the wind. It's a great fishing kayak because it's wide and stable and doesn't tip over at all (even when standing on it). But these good properties also make it like paddling a barge around - not very sleek. Let's put it that way.

Well, I made it back to catch the last of American Idol (country week - yuck) but instead of watching and relaxing I had to clean up that bluefish that I caught yesterday. I made quick work of it and then cooked up the striped bass fillet that I had taken out of the freezer in the morning. I took half of the bluefish and put it in the brine for smoking and the other half I will cook for breakfast tomorrow. Yum - bluefish and rice and beans for breakfast. (That was a sarcastic Yum)

I am looking forward to sushi lunch tomorrow. I need that because I don't have time to make lunch and it's a long day of work followed by my digital photography class - ending at 9 pm! It's my first time back to the sushi restaurant after giving them that nice striped bass so I'll let you know how that goes. I gave up my sushi lunch last week but not this week. I have been really good with my challenge lately and I deserve it. I also didn't use any Old Bay and this week's reward of flour, breadcrumbs and oil is not very exciting. I am going to have to re-think these rewards if I ever do this again. I think that big old chocolate brick would be a great week 2 reward because I could ration that and have just that little taste of chocolate every now and then. I think I may invoke the Special Occasion Reward in exchange for this week's reward so I'm not going to use any of the flour, oil or crumbs if I don't have to.

That's all for tonight - not too exciting. I have been looking at my daily body photo compilation to date. I have been very good about trying to take a photo at the exact same time and position every morning. So far, I don't see much visual change. I feel skinnier but I don't think it shows well in the photos. I will also compile my weight and blood pressure graphs and report that progress in the upcoming days.

DAY 17 - SASHIMI LUNCH

"There are two ways of spreading light - to be the candle or the mirror that reflects it."

~ Edith Wharton

It's tough to write stuff every day! So far, I've not much to report. My weight dipped a little bit again today (15 pounds lighter than the starting day). I feel quite good. I was really looking forward to my sashimi lunch but it was a bit anticlimactic.

The owner was very thankful for the fish that I gave him last week. However, he didn't give it to the sushi chef to use it in the restaurant. He brought it home and ate it in a variety of ways with his family. My regular sushi chef was not there today - replaced by someone else. Apparently he picked up a different job in New York and won't be back. That sucks because we had built up a nice rapport and he used to hook me up with a nice variety of sashimi that he didn't give to everyone else. He called it the VIP sashimi lunch. So today when I got the sashimi lunch, it came with all the basic fish and when I saw the new guy starting to slice some striped bass to give to me I had to protest! I asked him nicely to substitute another fish for that. After all, if I'm going to have this nice treat for myself for one lunch this week, I'm not going to get striped bass!

Overall it was good - but it was very similar to all of my meals lately - fish and brown rice. I did eat all of my daikon radish and kale so I got a little veggie in me as well. I could have gone overboard with one of the unique rolls and special sauce - but what I ate was the closest I could get to stay true to the spirit of the challenge. (I told you I've been good lately.)

Then the check came with no mention of "on the house" or "let me buy you a couple lunches" in exchange for the nice fish you gave me. Not that I was really expecting it but I was hoping for something. Something. I'm not totally disappointed - a little charity goes a long way. Although I didn't necessarily get anything tangible from them, perhaps in the future I will see the results of my act of kindness in another way that I can't even imagine today. We'll see. Maybe nothing. And that would be ok too.

As I was finishing up my day at work and getting ready to go to my photography class - my belly was quite full. I don't have much hunger at all - but I do want some junk/comfort food. There's a half of a chocolate angel food cake laughing at me about 20 feet away. I can hear it from here. It's faint, but if you're quiet and if you listen carefully, you might be able to hear it too. It's a little chuckle but it's definitely directed toward me.

DAY 18 – FORGETFUL

"From mistakes we learn. From successes - not so much. Keep moving forward."

~ Meet the Robinsons

Whoops! I had a little brain fart today and I forgot to prepare myself some breakfast AND lunch before work. It was an early start and I was checking e-mail or something and before I knew it I had to leave for work. I had a bluefish fillet in the fridge but not cooked and I had some rice and beans but I didn't pack any. I also had leftover greens that I am still a bit repulsed by. So needless to say, I had about an eight hour stint from 5 am on without anything but water (and that damn piece of left-over chocolate angel food cake staring at me - sitting in a Ziploc bag on the counter all day at work).

No, I didn't eat it. Interestingly, I was not feeling the hunger at all. I kind of like that. My cravings were minimal and it wasn't like I was dying to get some food in me.

This made me realize a pretty important thing about eating. I think the more that you eat, the hungrier you become. You start to get used to eating larger amounts and more frequently - and then that becomes the norm. And the times when you're not getting your feed bag on, you feel really hungry. This causes you to eat more - and then more and then more. The converse is true as well - when you start to condition yourself to eat less and less, your body doesn't give you the same cues to want to eat. In my case, the hunger and the need are not nearly as intense. I could take it or leave it and today when I didn't have any food in the whole first half of the day, I wasn't really bothered one bit.

I suppose that's how the starving people in the world eventually feel. For them, food is not really a high priority because they don't have the access to it like we do. Well, I'm not going to go off any more in that direction - that's another ball game.

When I got home I made a small meal from the bluefish, beans, rice and yes, even the dandelion greens. I stuck it in the toaster oven on some tin foil and set it to broil. Well, I got a little sidetracked and about 15 minutes later I could smell my meal burning up. I caught it in time for it to still be edible but it was a little on the extra crispy side. Oh well.

Later in the afternoon, Jamie got the idea in her head to make marshmallows. We do that from time to time so we typically have all the ingredients lying around. Corn syrup, gelatin, sugar and water are all you need. The two of us made a batch of marshmallows and it was VERY tempting to lick the bowl and the mixer with all that sticky gooey sugary whiteness. I watched the kids do it - and that was enough for me.

I'm planning on fishing in the morning because the striped bass reports are insane again but the weather report is for wind, wind and more wind. It's supposed to be nice and warm but the wind will make the sea very difficult for me in my boat. I'm going to brave through it though - I expect a little sea sickness and misery but I'm hoping to get in, get some fish and get out. I'll tell you how it all goes down.

DAY 19 - GREAT DAY FOR FISHING!

"Nothing will ever be attempted if all possible objections must first be overcome."

~ Samuel Johnson

I had asked several people to go fishing with me this morning - you know who you are! And ALL of them bailed out at the last minute or came up with some type of excuse - work, weather, doctor's appointment, communion preparation, etc. It was almost enough to make me not go. But all I can say right now is YOU ALL MISSED OUT.

The weather could not have been any better. The water was flat calm and no wind at all - thanks Mr. Weatherman for screwing up yet another forecast. I left at 6 am and I was around Sandy Hook and heading south to Monmouth Beach by 7:00ish. My fears of rough water and sea sickness and wind were all put to rest. The ocean was like a calm lake with no rolling waves whatsoever. The sun rising over the ocean was really cool.

It was just me by myself and I was hoping to catch three big stripers (two plus a bonus tag fish) to bring home with me. I had no bait - just jigs - so I was really on a hunting mission, looking for bird activity along the horizon. I didn't see any activity until I reached the area just off shore from Monmouth Beach. I don't know why this particular area has so much life all the time but it seems like boats, birds, bait and bass are all drawn to this spot. I started chasing down birds that I saw diving into the water and I was also looking closely at my fishfinder for signs of underwater activity.

The patches of fish and birds were very sporadic early on. The fish that were there were not biting the jigs I was throwing. I kept switching lures and trying new tactics. I had one on and then lost it. The second bite I had, I snapped my line at the reel (tackle/operator malfunction). A few times I was right in the middle of a school of feeding bass and I could not get them to bite. I could see all the bait in the water and these huge bass coming right up and swirling all around me. The water was calm and crystal clear so it was easy to see deep down. I can't tell you how many times I threw a lure right into the middle of a bunch of feeding fish without a bite. Very frustrating! There was just so much bait and food in the water that the fish were not interested in what I was tossing to them.

I switched my jig again to a smaller plastic storm shad (figuring this would more closely match the size of the baitfish) and that seemed to do the trick. I caught two small ones right away. Then for a long while the fish disappeared and I was back on a hunting mission. I travelled a LONG distance for my boat - all the way down to Manasquan and back. I could only do this because the water was so calm and easy to navigate.

I started heading back north figuring I would just continue to look for birds and signs of life and I would also start moving closer to home rather than further away. My gas supply was starting to worry me too. Running out of gas in the ocean is not an option for me to even toy with. Well, on my way back I saw this big flock of birds just sitting in the water. I rode over to check it out and they all scattered but what was just beneath them was a MASSIVE school of baitfish (rainfish). The birds knew it was just a matter of time before the predator fish would start to chase the bait to the surface. So I parked my boat in the middle of the school, shut off my engine and waited. It didn't take long as the first signs of big fish life started showing on my fish-finder. I tossed out my jig and hooked up immediately - and these fish were bigger than what I had been catching. All of a sudden there was an eruption at the surface - all around me. I wish that I had time to grab my camera to take a video because it was a spectacular site to see. But I was very busy making sure that I got my limit of fish before the whole thing was over. You never know how long something like this will last so you have to take every opportunity to catch the fish while they are there.

One after the other I was pulling in big stripers. They weren't huge, but all keeper size (over 28 inches). I had three rods with me so I would cast one out, hook up, and then put the hooked up rod in a rod holder and grab another rod to cast out. At one point, all by myself, I had three fish on at the same time. Luckily they didn't cross paths and tangle all the lines. What I like about this tactic is that I would keep these hooked up fish close to the boat and as a result it attracts the other fish to the general area. It was a way to keep the school around me for as long as possible. I wound up catching about six before the action died down. I was allowed to keep three because I have a bonus tag that I purchased online for $2. Well worth it.

Because of the gas situation and having my limit of fish, I decided to head home. It was only about 10:30. I didn't see any more life as I was driving back in so I just put the throttle down and zoomed home. Unfortunately, when I got back to the Shrewsbury River I got pulled over by the State Police! I was speeding. Go figure. Another boat was right next to me doing the same thing but he was just a little behind me so I got pulled over and he didn't. The cop gave me a warning and checked all of my credentials. It was mostly just a hassle but luckily he didn't give me a fine or a ticket.

My boat ran very well again - without a problem. I tested out my new livewell design and that seemed to work well too. I kept my fish alive right up until I pulled into my driveway and then put them on ice. I am going to have a little striped bass sashimi tomorrow for lunch I think. I will have a lot of fillet work to do but it's supposed to be 85 degrees and sunny so it should be a great day outside.

After I got home I had a handful of rice and beans (that's all I had to eat all day to that point by the way) and I got the smoker grill ready for the bluefish strips that were drying in the refrigerator. They took about three hours and came out very good. Again, I couldn't stop myself from eating it all up and now I don't have any for tomorrow. I cooked homemade pizzas for Debbie and the kids (they came out fantastic) using this dough I bought from a NY style pizzeria. There was so much leftover and I really wanted a slice (or five)!

I am really starting to get a craving for meat like a burger or a goose or maybe a little bunny rabbit. I got this idea into Ty's head and he's all for trying to trap a goose or a rabbit. I didn't go down that road last year at all but I have to be honest, I'm really thinking about it this time. I'll have to check out the 'legalities' of catching a wild goose or yard bunny before I start to make traps. But that's what surviving is all about. I have plenty of fish for a while and I am going to preserve it well in vacuum freezer bags so that it lasts a long time. But there's only so much fish I can take. I need variety to please my taste buds. We'll see.

Day 20 - Half Way Home!

Here we are at the halfway point - Day 20 - and still going strong! In a couple days I will have completed my third week and the reward for week three is fruit (a pineapple, orange and lemon). Debbie picked them up at Whole Foods today so that the pineapple would be ripe (hopefully) by Monday. This fruit is going to taste really good - especially the sweetness of the pineapple. I skipped my last weekly challenge reward because I am going to trade it for an upcoming Special Occasion Reward.

Carly's communion is next Saturday and Mother's Day is Sunday. Gary is having a party afterward at the Trump Country Club so there's no way I want to go there and not eat. I will be looking forward to that.

It feels good to be halfway done but there's still a lot ahead and it's not going to be easy. It has been most difficult getting greens to eat and I think I am lacking in that department - nutrition wise. Earlier I mentioned that a friend has a garden that she said I could raid to get some spinach and some other more common greens. I haven't done that yet but I'm considering it. It kind of compromises my rule system a bit so I'm hesitant. Speaking of rules, going through this for the second time has made me rethink some of my rules and rewards. I will have to remember for next time to put some type of green veggie reward in. I could leave out the Week 2 rewards of flour, breadcrumbs and oil. Although last time I fried up some fish - this time I don't really have the desire to do that. And nutritionally speaking, those items are not very helpful anyway. The fruit is good but won't last very long. I like the idea of a Week 2 BIG chocolate bar reward. But maybe that's just my sweet tooth talking.

Debbie had a good idea about a reward. For those of you who actually watch the show 'Survivor,' every once in a while they have a food auction. The players get to bid on certain food items and sometimes they are good but sometimes they are 'mystery' items and you don't know what you're getting until it is unveiled. Well, Debbie thought that it would be fun to make up three different dishes or food rewards, cover them and allow me to choose one. On the show, sometimes there are duds under the covers - like "You just bought a bowl of octopus brains for $200" so she was going to try to mimic this model. I don't know? It's an idea we were toying with.

Today I had a lot of striped bass to fillet so I got my station ready and went to work out in the yard. It takes time to clean these fish properly and the scene always attracts a group of kids from down the street. They love seeing all the guts and the head and inside the stomach to see what the fish had been eating. I give them rubber gloves so they can touch it all without getting any on their hands.

Today, the Buckman kids came over and we were all fascinated with fish brains and eyeballs and all the little fish that were partially eaten. Sounds gross but it's a great learning experience - especially for them to feel it all. They had so many questions about different organs and parts - things I didn't know. We're going to have to look these things up someday.

The eyeballs are particularly popular with the kids. They ask me to pop them out and cut them open and when I do I have them all touch it and feel what it's really like. Then when we cut it open (after all the goo explodes out and a group "ewww" is echoed by all) we found the hard, clear, marble-like lens that is inside each eyeball. It's actually pretty neat if you've never seen that before.

Except for Ty, all the other kids are grossed out by eating fish! I was shocked. I'm sure it's because they have never had it as fresh as it is here and as tasty as I make it. So, after cleaning the fillets I took a piece and sautéed it up in some butter with a little salt and pepper. Of course I had to bribe most of them to try it but once they did - they all liked it. I wasn't forcing it on anyone but it was so good and fresh and tasty that I promised a few of them that I would take them for a ride around the block in the bike-kayak if they just gave it a try. That seemed to work. After all, I'm just trying to broaden their horizons a bit. How can you be SO against trying a piece of fish if you've never had it before?

The ride reward was fun for a while but they wanted to keep going faster and going around the block over and over. Although I rationalized that this was good exercise for me (and it was) - enough was enough. It's tough enough riding my bike towing the kayak but add the weight of three kids and it's quite difficult.

Ok - back to Survivor. . .

For lunch today I fixed myself a nice little striped bass sashimi plate. I was very pleasantly surprised at how good it was. I really take care of my fish well and this is a testament to that fact. It was clean and fresh and quite delicious. Debbie's mom, Nancy, came over for a quick visit and her timing was perfect for sashimi so I sliced up a dish for her to have as well. Honestly, it was a lot better than I thought it would be and although it's a somewhat bland, white fish - it had a nice flavor of its own. We all enjoyed it - except Jamie who is strictly a tuna and salmon sashimi eater (for now).

Later in the day, Ty and I were still toying with the rabbit/goose idea. I found an old wrist rocket that I have had for years and we had some target practice in the backyard with a cardboard box. He's the perfect age (9) to get very excited about such a weapon. And yes, I am being as careful as possible and supervising at all times. After all, he may shoot his eye out.

Of course this attracted the attention of the young Buckman boys who were all too eager to have a turn. We had a lot of fun with this but ultimately I don't know if I'm at that stage just yet. Debbie is quite against it. We also saw two geese that would have been easy pickings down by the park today. I think geese always are in pairs with their mate so I wouldn't want to break up a pair. But, if the opportunity comes up and I see a lone goose who has lost its life partner, maybe I'll think about it some more.

More sashimi for dinner - and tomorrow I have to preserve all of my clean bass fillets in vacuum freezer bags for the future. I also set aside a bunch of strips and soaked them in some brine overnight so that I can get the smoker going again tomorrow.

Tomorrow is the NJ Shore Marathon and it is literally going past my front yard! We are basically trapped all day at the house because all the streets are being blocked off for the event. I'm sure it will be interesting though.

DAY 21 - MARATHON DAY

"The spirit, the will to win, the will to endure - these qualities are much more important than the actual events that occur."
~ Vince Lombardi

Don't misunderstand, this was not a marathon day for my Survivor Diet Challenge - it was the actual NJ Marathon and the route was planned to go right past our front lawn. What a neat experience. Thousands of runners went by from 9 am until 1pm. It was a hot 85 degree day and these people were sweating. We moved our sprinkler to the front lawn and pointed it into the street so the runners could go by and get a quick sprinkle of water. They were really appreciative and overall they were very nice people.

We were unable to go anywhere by car because the streets were all blocked off so the kids and I got on our bikes and went for a 'marathon' ride to see the finish line.

Before we left for our ride I had a nice plate of sashimi striped bass and a bowl of rice. I didn't think I'd be enjoying the striped bass sashimi as much as I have been but it is actually quite good. (Have I mentioned that already?) I have to admit that I have been using a tiny bit of soy sauce for dipping. Oh well - I don't feel too bad about 'bending' the rules a bit.

Afterward we went out to a little Italian restaurant for lunch. The kids were hot and stuffed their sweaty little faces with cheese steaks and turkey subs while I enjoyed a bottle of water.

We also took a trip to the BEST Italian Ice place in the world - Strollo's Lighthouse. Now this is a true test of will power for me. The line was long and I stood there watching all of these different combinations of flavors going by. The kids got soft ice cream. SOFT ICE CREAM??? At the best Italian Ice place in the world? Come on kids! Well, someday they will learn. Once again I just stood by and watched and put this place on the top of my list of places to go when I am finished with my challenge.

In the afternoon I started up the smoker again to do a nice batch of striped bass strips that I had been brining and drying for the last couple of days. It turned out well. I didn't eat much of it because I had so much sashimi bass and rice throughout the day. I just kept slicing off some pieces whenever I got hungry. It was so easy to prepare. I packed up the smoked bass and put it in the fridge - this will be a nice snack for whenever I need a flavor boost.

I'm doing pretty well with my rations of beans and rice so far. I'm past the halfway point of the challenge and there is just a little more than half left of rice and beans. Tomorrow I get to cut into that pineapple too - so things are looking up.

Dinner was more sashimi and rice and I actually made a plate up for Ty and Debbie - there was so much of it. I spent a good hour today vacuum packing striped bass pieces for freezing. I have a lot of reserves now. What I really need to cruise to the finish line is a little variety. Where will I find that?

DAY 22 - LUCKY MR. TURKEY

"Defeat is not the worst of failures. Not to have tried is the true failure."
~ George Edward Woodberry

I dropped off the kids at school today and in addition to the normal resident geese that I usually see on the school grounds, there was a wild turkey. The kids were very excited and wanted me to just go out and "get that turkey." I told them that turkeys don't want to be gotten and it wouldn't be as easy as inviting him over for dinner. Turkeys are really fast! Ty wanted me to go right back home and get the wrist rocket and some marbles and take some shots at this bird. I have to be honest - I really wanted to do the same thing. A wild turkey would make a fantastic meal and is just the variety I have been searching for.

Well, the only things I shot were a few pictures and a cute little video - this turkey was one lucky bird today! I disappointed the kids but Debbie told me that I would have some good karma coming my way as a result.

Oddly enough my weight went back up to 179 at this morning's weigh in. This was strange to me - but good. My goal is really for my BP to get as close to normal (120/80) as possible and I have definitely seen improvement in that since starting the challenge. Soon I will get around to compiling my photo log of my body which I have been taking each morning. I don't see too much change but I'm starting to hear from other people that I'm losing weight.

I ate my orange for breakfast - the whole orange - skin and all. I figured it would be nutritious even though it was quite bitter. I made it last all morning and thoroughly enjoyed the sweetness of the orange when I got to the inside. I carved up my pineapple very carefully and froze most of it so it would last a while. I scraped off every bit of fruit from the skin with my teeth and didn't waste a bit. It was perfectly sweet and ripe. Yum. It's been so long since I had a 'sweet' flavor that I wanted to gobble up the whole thing but I am going to be smart and ration it. The lemon - don't really know what to do with that yet.

I had a couple pieces of smoked bass throughout the day and for dinner I cooked some fish sticks, green beans and edamame for the kids and

Debbie and grilled some bass ribs for myself. I fixed my gas grill today and now it is working again. I think I had some spider webs in the Venturi tubes so I just had to clean them out. Apparently that is a common thing to have happen and now it has happened to me. Now I can advise people who have a malfunctioning grill and suggest that they may have "spiderwebs clogging up their Venturi tubes." Ha.

That's it for today - could have had a nice roast turkey dinner! I wonder how you clean a wild turkey? I think it's just a matter of time.

Day 23 – Reflection

"Not by age, but by capacity is wisdom acquired."
~ *Titus Maccius Plautus*

I have nothing significant to report today. Fish, rice, fish, rice, some greens here and there, some wild garlic and onions. Bad breath - and an occasional sweet treat of frozen pineapple. I do have some observations that I have been meaning to write about. It's just been so busy lately with the past few reports that I haven't shared some other insightful things that I have discovered during this experience. I think you may find it interesting too. . .

I was trying to compare my Survivor Diet Challenge to the challenges facing the contestants on the TV show, 'Survivor' and also to people in general who go on diets. In addition I want to share some thoughts on how my overall health has been altered by not eating 'convenience foods' and how people can make similar changes to their health (without having to get as extreme as a Survivor Diet).

Sometimes I envy the people on this show because there are tropical fruits (coconuts, mangoes, banana trees) and many varieties of fish, clams, crabs, and other sea life. Sometimes there are wild chickens. My point is that in the tropics, there 'seems' to be more variety available. Yet, in some ways the people on the television show have it more difficult than I have it. They don't have access to refrigeration, grills, various cooking utensils and the internet for information, etc. These are conveniences that the "suburban survivor" has. However, I believe that there is one very significant factor that I have to deal with - that they do not. That is WILL POWER.

Throughout this whole experience I have been very good - mostly honest and true to my rules. Every so often there is some little thing that I slip with - but really not much at all. My biggest challenge is having the will power to resist ALL of the other food and sources of food that are everywhere around me. The television Survivors don't have to deal with this because they don't have desserts and food and restaurants shoved in their face the whole time. That is incredibly difficult and is more of a mental game than anything else. Will power.

It is especially difficult on nights when I have to cook for my family and doubly difficult when my kids sit there and don't eat all of their vegetables or leftovers! Nobody in my family likes leftovers except me and I am usually the one to eat the leftovers the next day. Now our refrigerator is piling up with leftovers and all of this food is never going to be eaten. Every time I open the fridge it is packed with things to eat and I have to push it all aside to find my pot of brown rice or beans.

This is the dilemma that so many people face when they diet. Diets are utterly ridiculous! I am convinced of that. People can't possibly have the will power to stick to a diet plan when all of industrial America is against them. Fast food, advertisements, soda pop - not to mention the whole pharmaceutical industry. Don't even get me started on that one. Debbie got us to watch the television show, "Jamie Oliver's Food Revolution" over the past few weeks and admittedly I was hesitant at first. However, it is an eye opener to what 'Big Business' has done to the health, drug and food industries in America and this one guy is truly fighting a revolution. I highly recommend it for anyone who has not seen it. This guy has so much passion for a cause that is so RIGHT and he is met with resistance every step of the way. And I have to say, after watching several episodes, it all comes down to two things: money and ignorance. You can combine both of those things in a category of 'convenience' but money and ignorance are the culprits.

Money can be divided into 1) The money made by Industrial America's Big Business that keeps the machine perpetually going and growing. and 2) The money that people are not willing to spend on the better quality/less processed food items.

Ignorance is the general population accepting what has been done for years and years and not fighting to make a change - even at the great expense of their health and the health of their kids (and their kid's kids). Ignorance is not learning how to properly shop for and prepare your own meals but instead relying on the fast foods and convenience foods of today for the majority of your nutrition.

Sorry to go off on a tangent here. (This is what happens when I ask Debbie to write my log for a day - Ah, just kidding). Going through a Survivor Diet Challenge can open your eyes to these types of things and this is an opportunity for me to play my little part in the revolution. It may be a little extreme at times but my hope is that when I am finished with my 40 day challenge, I take some of what I have learned and apply it towards my future eating habits. Today I took my blood pressure and it was 118/88. That's a significant improvement from the start of this challenge. And that's only one of the measurable changes that I can quantify which shows that eating healthy, whole food is making a difference. You don't need to take medicine - let the food you eat be the medicine and your body will cure itself. That's all it does – it fixes itself. Headaches - gone. Weight - under control. BP - almost back to normal. It would be interesting to get a cholesterol check too - I know it was very high in the past but I don't have an exact point of reference to compare it to.

Let my experience be an eye opener for you (Mom). It doesn't mean you have to do my Survivor Diet (although it would be nice if some others did it with me!). What it means is that you need to take a step back, look at the big picture and join the revolution. If you have health problems of any kind, it's never too late to make a significant change and let your personal machine (your body) do what it does best. You just have to provide the right fuel. Don't be IGNORANT. Spend your MONEY on the right things. It may not always be the most convenient thing or the easiest - but it will be worth it in the end.

Day 24 - When the Challenge is Over

"If you want uncommon success, you must be uncommon."
~ Unknown

Sorry to be boring today but when you're at work from the early morning until 6 pm, then go to photography class from 7 to 9, there's not much to report. As much as everyone likes to hear about other people getting root canals, I'm not going to go there (yet).

I was smart this morning - cooked up a nice bass fillet with some salt, pepper and rice. I added some smoked bass and packaged it up to take to work. I snacked on it a little on the car ride, then again mid-morning, then again in the late afternoon and again between work and class. I just stretched it out to make it last. I did have my customary sushi lunch today. I don't know why but it still feels like I'm cheating when I do that. Maybe it's because I am - but like I said in the rules, if I don't have the time to 'survive' during the long work days, I need to incorporate this lunch into the system. Oh well - I'm not going to defend myself about that.

I still don't have any plans for that lemon - other than to sprinkle it on some fish?? That seems like a waste. A glass of lemonade would be nice but I have no sweetener. I have about a teaspoon of syrup left - that might work - all for one glass of lemonade? Not worth it. Actually, the orange and the lemon were somewhat of a waste of weekly reward I must say. So far my rewards have been kind of sucky - with the exception of the butter. That was the best reward yet. I am halfway through my second stick so I've been rationing that well since that first week of indulgence.

Hmmm. Let me think - next time around (if there is one) my first week reward will still be butter (and some quantity of peppercorns - that was a nice addition as well but I'm getting a little tired of pepper lately). The second week would be that brick of chocolate that I so often talk about. I could cut that into a thousand little bites and just suck on one every now and then to get the sweetness. Third week would be some type of vegetable buffet - maybe just a mess of greens to supplement what I am lacking most of all. We'll see how impressed I am with Week 4 reward (big juicy hamburger) when the time comes. And Week 5 is already an 'anything goes' - so how can you beat that? I think my chocolate brick may be arriving the Monday of Week 5!

I have been thinking lately about what I am going to revert to eating after my challenge is over. That's always a tricky time. If you watch TV's Survivor, you know that by the time they all get back to their lives on the mainland and do the final episode, everyone is back up to their original weight (and then some). The trick is to not let that happen. Especially with junk food and garbage and snacks between meals and desserts - Oh, that all sounds so good!

Well, it's time for another one of those questions to thy self:

"How can I continue to maintain a healthy, balanced lifestyle after the SDC and have fun in the process?"

My buddy Tony Robbins taught me to always add, 'and have fun in the process' at the end of these types of questions. That is the true question indeed. Everyone who has ever lost weight from a diet plan knows that what you do AFTER the diet is over really determines how successful you are.

Some ideas that I have been messing around with are:

- start some type of exercise program (yuck!)

- well, that's it so far.

Looks like I have some more pondering to do. I'll figure it out though.

Day 25 - More Boring Crap

"A ship in port is safe. But that's not what ships were made for. Sail out to sea and do new things."

~ Grace Hopper

I need to liven this challenge up a bit. Right now it's boring boring boring! Early start to today. I didn't have the desire to cook at 5:30 am, so I just stuffed a bunch of pre-cooked beans and rice into a lunch container and brought it to work. I sprinkled a little salt on it for flavor. Man - that salt is lasting a long time - that was a great idea to make the salt the first week. I use a tiny bit on almost everything.

I paid the price from lack of preparation at work today because all I had was. . .you guessed it, beans and rice. How much beans and rice can one person eat? Luckily I finish work at 2 pm. I have some defrosted bass in the fridge that I can cook up. I may even have some grilled bass in there too. I should have added that to my lunch box. Oh, and I did have a few pieces of frozen pineapple as I was getting ready for work this morning – that helped.

I haven't been doing too much active 'surviving' this week. What's up with that? "No active surviving. . ." Oooooo, Weeeeee, "What's up with that? What's up with that? What is uuuuuuppp with that?" If you don't watch SNL then disregard my attempt at humor in the last couple of lines.

I am going to pick a bunch of greens this afternoon and forage in my backyard. It's time to do that again. Maybe I'll check on my fig twig. And I think maybe, just maybe I am going back on the hunt this weekend for some variety meat. I haven't seen any bunny rabbits in my yard yet. I think that box with the target and holes might be scaring them away.

DAY 26 - A SUCCESSFUL HUNT!

"Expect the best. Prepare for the worst. Capitalize on what comes."
~ Zig Ziglar

The hunter in me came out today and I was on the prowl. Fortunately for me, I was successful. Unfortunately, it was still fish that I was hunting - rather than the turkey, goose or rabbit that I have been thinking about lately. I dusted off my wetsuit this afternoon and got all of my gear ready for spearfishing. It's been a couple of years since I have tried this (unsuccessfully) in New Jersey so I really wasn't too optimistic. However, with all of the striped bass activity lately off the beach, I thought it was worth a try. My hunch paid off.

I geared up and drove to Monmouth Beach. I carried my stuff over the rock wall and onto the beach. The tide was high and the water was a bit murky. This was going to be a problem. When I got into the 55 degree water the initial shock was quite harsh. It didn't last too long though - my wetsuit gives me full coverage and I can last for about an hour in water this cold without any negative effects. What bothered me most was the clarity of the water – or lack thereof.

Initially I started swimming right around the rocks but the water was too shallow. I could only see about one foot in front of my face. This was not good. I needed to go out to deeper water. This was pretty easy as the current took me right out there. It was the swim back that I was more concerned about. All of a sudden I was about 100 yards off shore so I had to be careful. I took a few practice dives to the bottom and at 10-12 feet the water was still too murky to see anything. I couldn't even see the bottom until I was almost face to face with it. I hate this kind of diving. So typical of the Jersey shore.

Well, I decided that I probably wasn't going to see any fish so I was going to use this experience to practice holding my breath and work on some relaxation techniques. I went out a little further which was about 18 feet of water. At this location I took a deep breath and started my descent. To my surprise when I got to the bottom the water column from about four feet down was quite clear - clear enough to spot any fish swimming by anyway. And sure enough, after sitting still for about 15 seconds a nice big striped bass came close to investigate. I was shocked to see it and I didn't have a very good angle on this fish. I took the shot in haste and missed high. It was moving away from me and I wasn't sure I would get another opportunity at a fish all day so I made an attempt. It wasn't a very smart shot - but sometimes you get lucky. Not this time.

As I got to the surface I could feel my heart pumping with excitement. There were actual fish here and I had a legitimate chance at getting one now. The clear water made all the difference. It took about three minutes to reload and then another two to relax at the surface. When I went down again, I waited for old Mr. Striper and sure enough another one came swimming by. This one was definitely keeper size and I was patient not to shoot too quickly. I lined up my spear and took my shot. PERFECT! Right through the head - I stoned it. In spearfishing terms this means that I hit a perfect shot that killed the fish instantly. No major body wound and no suffering. It just rolled over and that was it. Sometimes when you shoot a big fish and miss the kill shot, you have a pretty good fight on your hands to get it secured.

This was great news. The rest of the time I spent trying to swim back to shore against the current. I took a few more dives to try to find a really big one but the other fish I saw were all around the same size. I shot one more for my limit and then came in. In total I saw about eight nice fish, shot two and missed two. I had to swim past two fishermen on the rocks when I came in and they were pleased to see my catch because it gave them encouragement to know that there were many fish out there.

Spearfishing is one of my all-time favorite activities and having success so close to home without the use of a boat or kayak is fantastic. Ultimately I would like to rig my kayak to take in the ocean for spearfishing - maybe later in the season. Well, I have two more striped bass to clean tomorrow - not that I'm ungrateful but I am really loaded with bass now. I should have no problem finishing out my challenge with that - unless I get totally sick of it.

I had some bass ribs for dinner and just sautéed them in some butter - that's really all you need to make it taste great. I'm not sick of it yet. . .

Day 27 - Special Occasion Reward Day

"A storm starts when the first drop starts dropping but when the first drops stop dropping the storm starts stopping."
~ Dr. Seuss

I was wondering how I would ever work this quote (that I totally love!) into my daily log. But after reading it again (and again), it seems appropriate to this entry in a metaphorical way.

Today was Carly's communion and we were also planning to go to the Trump Country Club for a brunch celebration afterward. As per my rules, I traded in my Week 3 rewards for this Special Occasion Reward and put the challenge on hold this afternoon. I indulged my sweet tooth and caught up on some much missed greens and veggies. All in all I did a pretty good job at not going over the top crazy - I think.

I'll try to recall a quick list of my food choices:

Caesar salad, grilled chicken pieces, couple slices of bacon, bloody Mary, piece of pound cake, asparagus, lox, eggs Benedict, raspberries, strawberries, blackberries, blueberries, honeydew melon, slice of ham, taste of filet mignon, grilled zucchini, roasted red peppers, capers, chocolate milk, two Oreos, cheese cake, tiramisu, sliver of chocolate cake, mini éclair, water - that's all I can remember. Is that overboard? I felt full afterward but I didn't really feel like I gorged myself. On the ride home I was VERY sleepy and felt quite full indeed.

We'll see how I feel in the morning. That will be the true test to see if I pay the price of being a glutton I suppose. Will power! It was sooooo easy to just eat whatever I wanted without controlling portions or caring about calories or excess or fat, etc. But alas, it's back to the challenge tomorrow. And then two weeks to go. . .

Now go back and read that quote again – it might make more sense.

DAY 28 - FEELING ILL?

"To know what to do is wisdom. To know how to do it is skill. But actually doing it tops the other two virtues by far."

~ Unknown

Nope. I slept well, woke easy and didn't gain a pound. Go figure. The weather was total crap today - cold and windy. I spent a while cleaning the two bass I shot on Friday. They were sitting nicely in an icy cooler and cleaned up quite well - sashimi style.

I shared with Ty and Debbie and we enjoyed the fresh fish for lunch (and dinner). I brined a bunch of fish strips and we are going to try to make some jerky tomorrow in the food dehydrator. Also - I looked up a recipe for fish broth and took the fish bones and heads and fins and boiled them up in a pot. I might make some fish soup or fish chowder or just freeze the broth for later use in some other application. See - just when I thought I could do no more with striped bass I found a couple new recipes. It's quite the versatile fish. Fish broth - heads, tails, bones - Oh my!

The only negative effect from my food fest yesterday is that I got a taste of the good life and I don't want to give it up again. I REALLY want some tasty food today. If you remember from one of my previous entries, when I don't (or can't) eat the delicious food around me, I don't crave it or miss it all that much. But when you go off the wagon and start to partake in the goodies, it's like the start of a storm. Tough to shut off once it starts. That's the REAL challenge for me - and for anyone on a diet.

DAY 29 - JUST ANOTHER MANIC MONDAY

"Anyone who stops learning is old - whether you're 20 or 80. Anyone who keeps learning keeps young."

~ Henry Ford

For lunch I grilled up some bass rib sections. I pretended that I made two racks of baby back ribs. I gave them a generous basting of butter at the end of cooking and they actually turned out very good. I must sound like a broken record but if most people who catch striped bass took half the effort that I take in tending to their fish after they are caught, they would come to really enjoy many parts that normally get tossed away. The rib sections contain the belly meat and anyone who knows anything about fish parts should know that the fish belly contains the most fat. Just like fat in a hamburger, the fat in fish breaks down when cooking and adds an incredible amount of flavor to the meat. Bass isn't a very fatty fish (unlike salmon) but what little there is can be found in this belly meat around the ribs. Ok enough on fish anatomy.

I found a way to make very good use of my 'too salty jerky' tonight at dinner. I had a beautiful piece of bass to slice up for sashimi tonight and after I laid it all out on the dish I used my micro planer and I grated the jerky over the top of the slices. This was a fantastic idea I must admit. I actually created a great little seasoning to spice up the taste of the bass sashimi. It reminds me of a previously posted quote, "From mistakes, we learn. From successes, not so much. Keep moving forward." (That was from the movie *Meet the Robinsons* by the way)

The jerky grated very fine and looked like sawdust over the top. It added just a hint of concentrated fishy saltiness to the sashimi. If anyone knows what "bonito flakes" are, this was the striped bass equivalent. I'll certainly continue to do this for salty flavoring for many other dishes. I grated a bunch over my rice and it added a really nice flavor. To think I almost threw the whole batch out after tasting it in the morning. Eating it whole was almost inedible, but grated - it works!

I had to cook for the other guys tonight and I made grilled honey mustard chicken with grilled asparagus and artichokes. It looked and smelled soooo good. Ugh. The toughest times are when I have to cook, prepare and serve real food to the rest of the family.

I also gave Debbie a box of chocolate covered marshmallows on top of graham crackers as part of her Mother's Day gift. I bought it online from a place that claimed to have the world's best chocolate and marshmallows. Debbie and the kids have been enjoying them for days now. I wish they would just finish them up already.

I took a few more fish pieces out of the freezer in preparation for the upcoming long days at work. I have to be smarter and more prepared in the greens department though. Oh, I almost forgot - it's Monday and the end of Week 4. My Week 4 reward is a big juicy hamburger with all the fixings! Oh, I'm going to enjoy this. Ty wants to go to Five Guys but I think I'm going to go for a more upscale burger - maybe at a steak house or something similar. More research is needed. I don't want to waste this reward on a fast food joint. I remember a burger in San Francisco that was topped with a slice of foie gras. Now where could I find that around here? Maybe I'll bring my jerky and grate some on my burger. Ha.

DAY 30 - WOW! 30 DAYS SO FAR.

"Success consists of a series of little daily efforts."
~ Mamie McCullough

I am 75% done with my challenge. It actually goes pretty fast once you get into a groove. I have to admit, the fantastic striped bass season (so far) has been a HUGE help. I have not felt hungry yet. Many times it is not hunger but just the desire for something different or sweet or savory that is difficult for me.

My butter supply is still strong since I have been taking care to ration appropriately. I just started my third stick yesterday. My beans and rice supply is also looking good. I thought I was going to go through all of that very quickly but after about 20 days you start to lose the desire for the taste of rice and beans. I would say that I still have one third left by the looks of my containers.

My weight seems to have stabilized after dropping 15 pounds in 15 days. For the past week it has not moved more than a pound in either direction. More importantly, my blood pressure is almost at normal levels. That's really good. I still need to get the diastolic down a few more notches if possible.

For breakfast today I had some striped bass sautéed in butter and a few dandelion greens. I cooked up some more fish for lunch and mixed it with some crushed beans. And for dinner I had (you guessed it) more striped bass. Sashimi this time - sprinkled with some grated striped bass jerky and a side salad of violet greens that Debbie found in the yard for me. Wow - when I write it all out like that it sounds very repetitive. Did I mention that I need a little more variety? Man-o-man. Enough of the striped bass already. Well, I am out of the sashimi quality fillets (the kids ate the last of it for dinner last night - they had nine slices each and are really enjoying it). What's left is in vacuum bags in the freezer. And lots of rib sections too.

I don't have much else to say about Tuesday because I don't really do any Survivor-like things when I am at work. Sorry. Happy to be over the 30 day milestone! Keep on truckin!

DAY 31 - A LITTLE HEADACHE TODAY - YUCK!

"Effort is a commitment to seeing a task through to the end; not just until you get tired of it."
~ Howard Cate

While I was at work one of my co-workers spilled a bottle of monomer on the floor. For those who don't know what that is, it's a liquid that we mix with powder to make hard acrylic. It is very caustic and I am very sensitive to the odor - which permeates the entire office when it is spilled.

And it doesn't go away. I'm sure that my headache is a direct result of that monomer spill yesterday. Ugh - I hate that stuff. I just have to suck it up and get through it - without any Motrin. A long day at smelly work and then photography class tonight. Hopefully it will run its course and be gone by tonight. We'll see.

- A little bass jerky for breakfast.

- Sushi lunch.

- Seasoned bass in butter for dinner.

- Water, water, water throughout the day.

Not much else to report today. My log is a bit short during the week, huh? Last year I had horseshoe crab and eels to eat by this point in the challenge. This year the bass have provided more than enough protein for me. I may try some crabbing in the river this weekend - it may be time for the first crabs to start arriving. I haven't had thoughts of wild turkey or bunny rabbits for a while now.

DAY 32 - MEGABURGER!

"Don't wait for extraordinary opportunities. Seize common occasions and make them great."

~ Orison Swett Marden

As you may or may not know, my reward for surviving past Week 4 is a big juicy hamburger with the works. I've been thinking about this since Monday - trying to figure out the best place to go for my "best burger ever!" I've had some really good ones close by - Ichabods, Zacharys, Barnacle Bills, The Pour House, Where's the Beef, Mudville Pub, KJ's, etc. All top notch by burger standards. But how was I going to top them all? Hmmm, where to go indeed? And then it hit me. . .

It was simple - I was the answer to my own question. Who could construct a better burger with everything I love on top and all around it? Nobody. It doesn't exist - except for in my own mind. So I was the logical choice to make . . . MEGABURGER! Little did I know at the time that this little project of mine would consume an incredible amount of my time and resources - so much in fact that I tried to compile a photo montage of my exploits.

You won't want to miss the upcoming megaburger log . . .

Two Days later . . .

It took a little time but I think it was worth it. If you're a non-beef eater reading this then you may not want to continue. Otherwise, I hope you enjoy it as much as I did. . .(not possible).

It's tough to really get the full effect of Megaburger without a detailed description of what went into its construction:

- The bread - Aleo's Italian Deli has long hard rolls that are amazing. What could be better? And I found one that was square-ish shaped. Perfect for megaburger. I sliced it open, extracted most of the inside, sautéed the inner bun in butter and then tossed it on the grill for some marks and some flavor.

- The beef - Originally I was shooting for an 80/20 mix for the perfect burger fat content. However, the quality of the beef is also important. I went to Whole Foods because I knew I wanted to get Cave Aged Gruyere cheese (more on that later) and in the butcher section I found grass fed beef. Yes it cost about double, and it was 85/15 but this was Megaburger and worth a little extra. To compensate for the lack of fattiness, I also got a half pound of ground lamb to mix in with the ground beef. A perfect combination. I gently mixed in some extra virgin olive oil, kosher salt and fresh ground pepper into the beef/lamb blend. I had enough for megaburger and two extra patties for the kids.

- Cheeses - Megaburger is stuffed internally with a big chunk of blue cheese. Then, at the end of cooking I sliced a slab of Gruyere and melted that over the top. Did I mention it was cave aged?

- The Works - Caramelized sweet yellow onion, sautéed portobello mushroom slices, sliced avocado, sprouts, a beauty of a slice of tomato, a scoop of chutney (consisting of yellow mango, lump crab meat, diced onion, avocado and tomato with kosher salt), romaine lettuce and special sauce (a blend of mayonnaise, ketchup, Worcestershire sauce and Grey Poupon mustard).

- The Sides - The perfect fries. These, I did not have the desire to make when I knew a trip to Five Guys was all I needed to do. They slice their potatoes on site and deep fry them not once, but twice to give them the perfect crispiness. The homemade equivalent just wouldn't do justice. I also grabbed some ketchup and malt vinegar while I was there. A side Caesar salad and a fresh sliced deli pickle rounded out the sides. (A layer of fries went between the bottom bun and burger as well).

- The Beverage - Wow, this was a no brainer. What is the perfect beverage to go with a megaburger? A Guinness, of course. A match made in heaven.

Well there you have it. No ordinary burger. I have to admit, I didn't finish it all in one shot. I needed a couple breaks along the way. But as Adam Richman (from Man v Food) would say, "In this epic battle of Man versus Food, today. . . Man was victorious!

DAY 33 - THE BASS GET BIGGER

"It takes courage to break through barriers and to go places you've never been before."

~ Anaïs Nin

The weekend weather outlook is good for fishing and outdoors. Finally. I worked most of the day and was done around 2:00 so I decided to check out the Monmouth Beach Surf Cam online. I use this frequently to see how calm or rough the ocean is. The wind was minimal and the waves were small so I started making plans to do some fishing. Next I checked the local tide chart to see what I would be dealing with. It was dead low tide. Not good for surf fishing.

I had to switch gears and come up with another idea. Debbie had to leave the house at 5 pm to go to the movies with her mom so my window of opportunity was slowly closing. The answer - an hour of spearfishing. I got all of my gear ready and was in the truck by 3:00 with specific instructions to be back by 4:45. I was in the water by 3:15. The best part about spearfishing here is that I can be in the water in 15 minutes. To get to the same location by boat would take about two and a half hours and cost about $40 in gas (in the best conditions).

My first dive was in about 13 feet of water (about 100 yards off shore) and visibility was terrible. My spear tip actually hit the bottom before I could see the bottom. Yuck! Not a good sign. I had to go deeper to see if I could find some clear water. I got out to about 18 feet on my next couple of dives and just by chance I found a great location. I found myself on a large area of structure - rocks covered with muscle beds, star fish, sting rays, horseshoe crabs, etc. It's really amazing how life underwater flocks to any area with structure. I grabbed some rocks to hold myself to the bottom and lay very still. The stripers didn't take long to show up.

My breath hold is still not up to par since this is only the third time diving in five years. The chill in the water (48 degrees - Brrr!) also makes it difficult to stay under for very long. My best bottom time for this entire trip was only 48 seconds. Most of the time it was somewhere between 25 and 40 seconds. When the stripers started showing up I was trying to be very selective. I didn't want to shoot any questionable fish so I was determined to let any small ones swim by and wait for the big ones to show. However, ALL of the fish I saw were in the 'keeper' size range (about 30 inches give or take two inches). It was difficult to watch these fish go by but I really wanted to go for a personal best. Currently my biggest striper is 35 pounds and that was a long time ago. There have been recent reports of 40+ pounders nearby so I knew there was a chance.

I was able to position myself to continually dive back to this structure area even though it was not visible from the surface. I started seeing some large blackfish and considered taking one of them home for supper. I passed on them after a particularly large school of stripers came into view. Or, I should say a school of particularly large stripers came into view. I held my breath and watched some 20 pounders swim past. Just as I was about to surface, a really big one came swimming past me to the right - significantly larger than the surrounding fish. It was time to take my first shot. I didn't have the best angle on this one but I was running low on air and needed to take the shot soon. I reached out, pulled the trigger and could clearly see my spear shoot high - just over the fish's head. Damn! On my way back to the surface I was livid. I belted out a bunch of underwater profanities and I was hoping that my missed shot hadn't scared the whole school away. Sometimes this happens. The vibrations of the shot going off can spook all the fish in the area and sometimes you don't see another one in the area for a long time.

It took me a while to reload and just as I was finished I looked down and saw a bunch of nice sized fish swimming right below me. I considered taking a shot from above but that is not a high percentage shot. I dove down and spooked a bunch of fish but gradually settled to the bottom and they curiously came back around. Not as big as my missed fish (of course) but I saw a few nice ones and picked one out to shoot. It wasn't the best shot but it did the job. I usually try to shoot for the stoning shot or a head shot but this one went through the body and will affect some of the meat. At least the fish were still there.

I was getting cold and I only had about three or four more dives in me so after stringing my fish up on my float I went back down with the mindset of not shooting again unless I saw something REALLY big. I lost my bottom structure because I drifted a long distance while I was at the surface. I also had a pretty long swim back to the beach and I was quite cold. But the fish were still there and you never leave fish - right? I took a couple more dives and watched a lot of 20 pound plus fish go by. But nothing that was standing out above the rest. On my way back in I managed to shoot one more fish that was in the same class as the first one. Then it was time to start swimming.

Both fish were 37 inches long. Both shots were far from perfect - but got the job done. It's nice to know that there's still a plethora of big bass right off shore and they are getting bigger. I'll get my personal best soon I'm sure. Just gotta keep on truckin.

Day 34 - Relaxing Saturday

"We all have possibilities we don't know about. We can do things we don't even dream we can do."

~ Dale Carnegie

I have been living off megaburger for the past two days. I haven't really felt hungry after eating that whole thing. Maybe that's my body's way of regulating itself. I've only been picking here and there on some rice and a handful of beans every so often.

Today I had to clean those two big fish that have been sitting on ice.

It's time to start giving some fresh fish away. I have plenty - I kept a couple of nice sections for sashimi and gave some really nice pieces away to some neighbors and friends. At around 3:00 pm I cooked up a small batch of fish scraps in butter with some salt and pepper and had a nice meal of it with some brown rice. I also took a bunch of strips and have it sitting in brine for the smoker. I will NOT forget to rinse this batch off I assure you.

Other than that - not much was happening on the Survivor Diet front today.

The kids had baseball/softball all day today. The weather has been perfect. I'm planning an ocean excursion with Dad tomorrow - in search of my record breaking bass. I'm bringing my wetsuit with me just in case the situation looks good for a dive. It should be flat calm all day based on the weather reports.

Day 35 - A Day Out With Dad

"You may be disappointed if you fail, but you are doomed if you do not try."
~ Beverly Sills

The weather report was a little off for today but Dad and I had planned to go out fishing so we did. It was a long and arduous boat ride to the Shrewsbury Rocks from my house. Took about two hours - remember I was complaining a while back that I can drive to the beach and jump in the water in this same location in 10 minutes??? Well, I should have done that instead. It was really great being out in the open air with Dad but we didn't have much luck with the big bass like I had hoped. It was too chilly to jump in the water to try any spearfishing. We got a couple nice reads on the fish finder but no bites.

When we decided to pack it in and head home we stopped to fly fish in the Shrewsbury River and right away we started catching a bunch of small bluefish. It was a good capper on the day. The sky was really cool looking with the cloud formations. I took some photos and a little video clip so Dad could do a little Stripping Guard promotion (www.strippingguards. com). I kept four bluefish to eat and we headed home. All in all it was a nice day to be outside and although we didn't get our BIG fish, I had already stashed enough fish away to last a while longer.

Since I'm doing shameless promotions for family members, this might be a good time to put a word in for Debbie's book - a healthy eating cookbook - which can be found at nourish-to-flourish.com.

Day 36 - Amazing Surf Fishing - M.B.

"Procrastination is the thief of time."

~ Edward Young

Not so much a Survivor post - but a great fishing report. I suppose they are one in the same these days.

I was moping around today wondering what to do. I knew I should go to the beach to check it out but I was just procrastinating. I fished all day yesterday and felt like I wasted so much time. And I didn't feel like suiting up in all of my gear for spearfishing. I checked the beach-cam and it looked so beautiful - should I stay or should I go? Well, I think I made the right choice to go.

The water was flat calm at the Monmouth Beach surf today at 1:00 pm. Except for the fact that it was BOILING as far as the eye could see with HUMONGOUS fish.

The largest was 42 inches and an estimated 30 pounds. In addition there were bluefish that measured 35 inches and an estimated 20 pounds! It was truly amazing and lasted for a couple hours. There was one other guy there and he was fishing with bait. I had it all to myself. Because of my recent success with so much fish, I did what was right and threw all of my fish back to bite another day. I must have caught 10+ bluefish all in the 15-20 pound range (this is unheard of for bluefish - they were the largest bluefish I had EVER seen) and two really nice bass in the 25-30 pound range. All fish were caught on a big, cheap ass, metal spoon (Krocodile imitation - $3 at K-Mart) and the largest bass was caught on a sand eel plastic with a wire leader. So much for bass being leader shy. Best day surf fishing ever.

DAY 37 - STUPID, JERKY

"Success is not final, failure is not fatal: it is the courage to continue that counts."

~ Winston Churchill

I can tell that my mind is starting to fall out of survival mode. There is light at the end of the tunnel and with three days left I am not being as prepared as I should for the finish. For example, today is my long day at work and I have a lunch break in the middle of the day. I NEED to plan ahead for Tuesdays and prepare some type of lunch or snack or meal for after work. I totally spaced out and forgot to do that today.

I have a freezer full of beautiful fish fillets vacuum sealed in individual portions - just waiting to be defrosted for meals. But I physically have to take them out ahead of time in order for them to be ready to prepare. Didn't happen.

I have four bluefish sitting in a bag in my refrigerator - ready to be cleaned. Didn't happen. See - that's what I mean about my mind starting to fall out of survival mode. Not a good thing. I know there's only three days left but I have to stick with it and not slack off.

The good thing is that a couple days ago I cleaned a few nice sized bass that I hunted and although I gave a lot away to neighbors and friends, I made jerky with the rest. I rinsed it off really well after brining overnight. Then I smoked it on the grill with apple wood chips for a few hours. After the smoking, the pieces were still quite moist. They were done, but too moist. These pieces of smoked fish would not preserve very long - even in the refrigerator. So I got out the dehydrator and put all of it in and let it go overnight. (Did I tell this story already? Sounds familiar.)

Anyhoo - I was afraid that the dehydration process was going to really overdo it if I left it out all night long. I was kind of right - when I checked it the next morning the pieces were very hard and a dark brown color. It looked surprisingly just like beef jerky. I tasted a piece and hoped that it would not be overly salty. It was not. And not only did it look like beef jerky, it tasted JUST like beef jerky! Pretty amazing. I bagged up the batch and put it in the fridge to be used another day. Today was that day.

I filled a small Ziploc with jerky, put it in my pocket, and there I had a nice snack whenever it was needed throughout the day. I drank a lot of water today too. Every now and then I would break off a piece of jerky and chew on it a bit to release the flavors within. I love beef jerky and this stuff is spot on quality beef jerky tasting - except it's made out of striped bass. Interesting huh? Well, my point is that my laziness and stupidity and lack of preparation for today's meals was salvaged by the jerky that I had previously made. And that took A LOT of time and care and effort to prepare. So I guess I am still surviving pretty well - tough to go a whole day on fish jerky and water though.

I have been giving more thought to how I am going to continue after my challenge is finished. I'm not going to go back to my normal eating habits - that would be stupid. I was thinking about my weekly rewards and how I look forward to them each time a new one is due to come up. I think it would be a good idea to continue to have a weekly reward - one. Something that I can plan in advance and that way there would be something to look forward to. I would still have to rely on my will power to not let it get out of control. That's the key. Will power.

In addition, I have been thinking about something called 'Seasonal Eating' which involves eating only the types of food that are currently available in the particular season you are in and in the region or parts of the world that you live in. It's kind of an extension of the Survivor Diet but allows for more freedom of choice and variety. For example, eat tomatoes when they are ripe and in season (late summer). Do not eat them at other times of the year just because your supermarket can have them shipped from Argentina or somewhere else where they grow.

I don't know a whole lot about this subject but what I do know makes sense to me. Because the SDC is purely a whole food, seasonal diet - I think it would make a great transition for when I finish. I still have a few details to work out.

My other idea for when I am finished is to make another challenge for myself - to try to get a ripped six-pack of ab muscles. I've only had that once (in college for a brief while before the beer took care of it) and since I have slimmed down significantly in the belly region, this may be the best and only time to start a challenge like that. I just have to think about how I can have fun in the process.

It seems like the only way to get those abs would be to do some traditional exercises that target those muscle groups. Maybe there is another way. Hmm. If I could figure that one out I could be a millionaire. It's good to know that I have a few more projects in the works after this challenge is over.

DAY 38 - THE V BRICK

"Believe me, the reward is not so great without the struggle."
~ Wilma Rudolph

I was very moody and stressed today. Mostly because of other things going on with work and banks and mortgages and slow-ass computers and speeding tickets and lawyers and broken windshields and rental cars and auto body repairs - blah, blah, blah, blah blah! You throw hunger on top of all that and you have the perfect recipe for moodiness and stress. Man I could go for a peanut butter cup.

It's totally true that stress in your life causes you to want comfort food - mostly sweets and junk food. I haven't craved much of anything throughout this challenge. Well, nothing that almost drove me to the brink of cheating. Until today that is. I wanted chocolate - and I wanted it badly. Soooo close to the finish line and I felt my will power draining out of me. I tried to fill my need with a few pieces of bass jerky. But guess what happens when you throw 'salty' on top of a comfort food crave? Yeah, you got it . . . the brain just wants to put something sweet on top. I could have eaten a gallon of chocolate ice cream.

So what did I do, you ask? What good is the Internet if you don't use it for some indulgence every now and then? In a matter of five minutes I found my 'end of challenge' prize. Enter The Valrhona Chocolate Brick. I've talked about this in the past but last week when I went to Whole Foods for my burger ingredients I found out that they didn't supply these chocolate bricks any longer. I was pissed. Not anymore. UPS is going to deliver my $42 brick of chocolate in two days. Oh yeah. Knowing that it's on its way is enough for me to stop the sweet cravings and go on with my day. After I ordered it, I didn't have to think about junk food any longer. (For anyone else who wants to take the shortcut to chocolate bliss – look up the Valrhona Chocolate Brick online.) OK, enough on that.

I snacked on jerky throughout the day. A handful of beans every once in a while. Water, water, water. Some sautéed bass in butter with salt and pepper for a late lunch. And dinner, well - who's got time for dinner? Poor planning once again made me miss dinner. Kids had gymnastics and baseball, I had photography class, got home in time to see who got kicked off Idol and that was it. I caught the aroma of the taco dinner that Debbie made for the kids when I walked in the door. I am much more sensitive to smells now. Interestingly, I am not hungry and I talked about this in a previous post. I think my body has gotten used to less food on a daily basis and I really don't feel the need or desire to eat too much. That's good and bad. Bad because I really don't know what's going to happen when I'm done.

Just as a side note, for photography class I took a really cool picture of a dragonfly on a flower. One of my cats actually captured the big bug and was torturing it. Mostly dead, but still very colorful and fully intact, I artificially propped it up on a flowering plant and snapped a few photos that came out really nice.

No, I didn't eat it! Haven't gone down that road. . .yet. Gonna try some crabbing tomorrow (maybe).

DAY 39 - BLUE CRAB FEAST

"A person who leaves nothing to chance does very few things wrong. However, he also does very few things."

~ Unknown

Ok - so I ruined the surprise with the title. And YES - tonight was a celebration of the first haul of Blue Crabs this season! It couldn't have come at a better time. Variety is the spice of life and my spice tonight was blue crab. It was so good and so sweet and I added a little drawn butter to kick it up to the next level. With fresh crabs you don't even need butter because they are so tasty by themselves - Mmmm, so good. Day 39 was awesome! But it didn't start out that way. . .

After some bass for breakfast, I took a quick drive to the beach in the morning to check out the surf. It was fairly calm but the tide was too low to fish very effectively. However, on my way there I crossed over the Monmouth Blvd. Bridge and I thought I noticed some bunker splashing way out in the distance. I thought to myself that today may be a better day in the river than in the ocean.

After the ocean was a bust, I trailered up the boat and dunked it into the river. I headed over to Branchport Creek to try to locate the schools of bunker. For those of you unfamiliar, bunker are baitfish that spawn this time of year in the upper branches of these saltwater rivers. They form massive schools and are a favorite food to many predatory species in the area. They also make great crab bait because they are very oily and have a strong scent which attracts everything to them.

It didn't take long and before I knew it I was smack dab in the middle of bunkerville. I used this opportunity to try out my new cast net. This is a large round net that you toss out like a giant Frisbee. It has weights all around the circumference and as the weights sink, anything underneath the net when it was tossed will get scooped up. It takes a lot of practice but I got the hang of it last year after watching some instructional YouTube videos. The new net is HUGE though - much more difficult to toss, and a whole lot heavier. I practiced throwing it for a while in the backyard last week and before long I was doing quite well.

The trick today was finding the bunker and then motoring up to them before they disappeared. It's tough to do when you're alone. I had some success. On my first few casts I picked up one or two here and there. Then I had a great toss on a close up school and hit pay dirt. It's possible to get a hundred of these fish in one toss if you are good. In this toss I probably picked up 20 or so. Not bad at all. I put all of the bunker into my homemade livewell and kept at it for about an hour. In total I must have netted about 40 fish. I tried to keep them alive as long as possible but when the tank starts to get over crowded there isn't enough oxygen to go around.

After getting as much bait as I could, I anchored the boat in the middle of the bay and thought I would take a chance at some crabbing. It is WAY early in the season for big crabs but with everything else that has been going on, you never know. I cut up a few bunker, attached them to three drop-lines and threw them over the side. While I was waiting for crabs I decided to send a live bunker out on a hook to see if anything would take it.

It wasn't long before the action started happening. I started pulling up my drop-lines and then looked over at my fishing pole which suddenly bent over with line screaming off the reel. I was hooked up with a very large bluefish. I wasn't using a wire leader so I was amazed that I was able to land this fish without breaking the line. It was huge (by bluefish standards) - about 12 pounds I would guess. I kept him for the smoker.

The action continued with the bluefish biting every few minutes and pulling up blue crabs in between. I was all by myself going nonstop for a couple hours. A lot of fun. I only had one throwback crab. All the rest were really big - already. This is a REALLY good sign for things to come. Lots of crabs, lots of bait, lots of fish around. I only kept the one big bluefish and tossed back about 4 others. I ended the afternoon with 15 nice crabs and one bluefish. And to think - I was only going out there to see if I could get some bunker for bait for tomorrow's fishing trip.

It just goes to show that you have to get out there and do stuff - you just never know what's going to happen, but if you don't ever try then it is certain that nothing will happen. I was a little dejected after seeing the beach in the morning but wound up having about four hours of excitement and fun by just getting outside and trying something new today. That's what the Survivor Diet Challenge is all about my friends!

Doing new and different things keeps your mind active, your attention alert and your body young and full of life. I can't tell you how many times I have set out to do one task and just by chance another opportunity crossed my path. One which I would have never known about had I not been out there doing things. Hopefully the kids of today (including my own) will get this message and look up from time to time from their phones or devices to see the world around them.

DAY 40 - THE GRAND FINALE

"A great pleasure in life is doing what people say you cannot do."
~ Walter Bagehot

I have been holding onto this quote – waiting for the final day.

Here we are - at the finish line. 40 days. I did it! I know, I know - you're all soooo proud of me aren't you? Well, I don't know who has really been reading this but for all you naysayers out there I just want to tell you that IT CAN BE DONE. And it's not as difficult as you might think. Here's a little recap of the challenge, a log of today and my plan for what is to come.

Today I was invited out with Pat to do some fishing (surprise - huh? more fishing). Well, it's always a pleasure to go out with Pat on his boat. He's a great host and a great guy all around. His boat is amazing and it gets us out into the ocean in a fraction of the time it usually takes me. I just wish that he didn't bring along the bag full of mini chocolate covered donuts! Thanks Pat! I still remember the chocolate covered strawberries a few weeks ago.

We had a bushel of clams and a load of bunker (alive and dead) and we were very optimistic about the adventure to come. It was a beautiful flat calm morning and everything seemed perfect except for the fact that the fish were not cooperating. We spent several hours riding up and down the coast for miles searching for signs of life but it just wasn't happening. On our way back in we stopped at Romer's Shoal and anchored up to do some bait fishing with clams. It took a while but our friend, Chick, eventually hooked up with a very nice sized striped bass.

This fish was 37 inches long. A very nice specimen indeed. Initially I thought that the size of this one topped the two that I caught on the beach the other day but my fish measured 42 inches. I still think that there is a 40 pound plus striper out there just waiting for me. It's going to be on my spear though - not my fishing pole. Maybe next week sometime if the weather is nice.

Ok - so Day 40. This is the final day of the SDC and for meals I had rice, bass jerky, and a lot of crabs. With the crabs, I couldn't have asked for a better final two days' worth of meals and activities. I enjoyed them better than anything that I could have bought or ordered in a restaurant. The final two days were not much of a challenge at all - they were a treat.

My beans, rice and butter rations held out well. I still have close to a stick of butter left and plenty of beans and rice. Admittedly, I got a little tired of cooking and eating beans and rice (especially beans). I think the main difference between this year and last was the fact that the striped bass came in and were so plentiful. I went back and read some early log entries and forgot how difficult it was for me and Ty to catch fish in the beginning. I can't believe that I was eating those little crappy sunfish from the pond down the road. It makes me feel better that Mr. Fredrickson was released back into the wild.

I would have liked to expand into small mammals or birds this time but other than that encounter with the turkey, I really didn't pursue it too aggressively. I had all the fish I needed so it kept my hunger under control. I was a little lacking in the greens department but today and yesterday I had a little 'wild green leaf surge' which I felt pretty good about. And by that I mean 'I ate a bunch of weeds from the backyard.'

Overall, I lost about 18 pounds! And my blood pressure seems to be very close to normal. I still need to get that down a bit. I don't think I really needed to lose that much weight but it will be no problem putting back on that last five pounds. I am happy with my weight and my small gut at the moment and I fit into some of my tee shirts and older dress pants a lot better. It doesn't look like I have a beer belly any longer. With tennis starting soon, I may be able to stay in pretty good shape over the summer. (I have to figure out a way to compile the photos of myself changing over 40 days.)

The question on everyone's mind . . . where do we go from here? I can't just end here because we need to know what happens next. Am I going to pig out tomorrow? Am I going to start that exercise routine to get my six-pack abs? Am I going to try to eat seasonally? How much weight is coming back on and how quickly? Will I ever get a shot to be on the TV Survivor??? Ha! Maybe someday. Jeff Probst, if you're reading - Come on man, give me a chance!

My initial plan is to eat seasonally, have a "reward" indulgence meal or special treat once per week, and spend two weeks on the P90 Ab Ripper X. I may overindulge tomorrow as a celebration but after that I'm not going to go too crazy. There are some chocolate covered marshmallows on graham crackers still around (I can smell them) and I think one has just been invited to breakfast. Ha.

Thanks for reading everyone. If anyone was inspired by my adventures/ misadventures and would like to join my SDC in the future, I would love to have some company. I will probably start in April each year.

In addition to my Dad's life motto of *"Never leave fish,"* I have another quote for the final day of my Survivor Diet Challenge:

"Sometimes you have to jump off the cliff and make your wings on the way down."

~ Ray Bradbury

Day 1 AD - Oh How the Mighty Have Fallen

"Greatness is primarily bravery to escape old ways and customs."
~ Unknown

My plans of not going overboard went overboard thanks to Rob and Monika's family birthday party for their daughter Amanda. It was a food fest and the desserts just kept coming. This came AFTER the personal delivery of an entire box of chocolate covered strawberries from Pat (Thanks again for that Pat!) in the afternoon. I completely gorged myself on chocolate covered strawberries - I just couldn't contain myself. Then at the party, well, I couldn't be rude. . . with all of those homemade desserts. It's going to be VERY interesting how my body reacts to this in the morning.

I started my first day AD with a delicious omelet stuffed with blue cheese and crabmeat - so good.

Later, we had a group trip planned to go strawberry picking at an organic strawberry farm. This was a lot of fun but instead of picking, I just did a whole lot of eating. I filled myself up on strawberries, which would most definitely qualify as survivor food because I was eating them right off the plants. They were amazing. Sweet as can be.

Debbie brought home about five pounds of berries and then when we got home, that's when Pat arrived with a big box of the chocolate covered. . . strawberries. I couldn't stop myself! So good.

Can you tell I have a little chocolate problem right now? In the afternoon the birthday party came and although I tried to have some self control, I just couldn't. One day after the SDC ends and I go completely sugar happy. You would have too if you saw the spread. I mean really - these cupcakes were homemade with little individual sugar coated marshmallow swirlies on top.

I'm not even going to reveal all of the other stuff I ate but I'm sure I will be paying the price very soon. See, that's why diets suck - because there's always an end. And when it ends, it's a free for all. There HAS TO BE A PLAN IN PLACE for the end. If not, then don't even bother. So I'm going to treat this little food fest like a 'weekly reward' in the SDC. I don't know if anyone noticed but I did not take my last weekly reward which was basically a pot luck - any meal I wanted. When I caught those crabs, well, that was the meal I wanted. So the reward was not necessary. (I think I'm trying to justify my actions.)

I'll try to be better from now on but with a fridge full of chocolate covered strawberries and a Valrhona brick on its way, I'm not making any promises.

Day 2 AD - Ab Ripper X

"Growth demands a temporary surrender of security."
~ Gail Sheehy

Well, other than the broken scale, I feel quite normal this morning. I slept like a rock. Passed out at about 9:00 pm with all of my clothes on and didn't move a muscle until 8:00 am. I was OUT. I guess a couple glasses of sangria had something to do with that after not having any alcohol for 40 days. But no headache, no hangover, no bloated yucky feeling in my belly - just nine extra pounds. How could that be? I mean, I admit that I went a little strawberry happy and I did have a few of those pizza bagels, and that hot dog, oh and that Polish kielbasa, the potato chips, a huge cupcake, a wedge of ice cream cake, perogies, salad, chocolate chip cookie, the crab omelet, a couple of s'mores, and sangria - but if I weighed all that stuff it still wouldn't equal nine pounds of food. Whatever. I'll see what happens tomorrow.

This afternoon I made my first attempt at exercise with the P90X system. I also had a couple chocolate covered strawberries and finished the last of the crabs. Anyway - I figured I would start with the Yoga X for 30 minutes and then see how much of the Ab Ripper X I could complete.

I have never done Yoga before so all of the moves were foreign to me. The tough part was doing the exercises and trying to watch them on the screen at the same time in order to get the form correct. I'm sure that after doing this pretty regularly, the terminology will become common to me. It's just going to take some getting used to in the beginning. All in all the Yoga X was manageable. It's a 90 minute routine on DVD but I started slowly with 30 minutes.

Then came the Ab Ripper X. Are you kidding me? This is only a 15 minute workout. I think I managed to actually do 3 or 4 minutes total - and that's just an estimate. If I can come back to this blog at some point in the future and report that I was able to do the whole 15 minutes of Ab Ripper X then my life shall be complete. This challenge is going to put the Survivor Diet Challenge to shame. I was so happy to hear the instructor say at the very end of the session, "Don't do this routine every day." I think that's the only instruction that I'm going to be able to do really well on the entire Ab Ripper X routine.

Now I have a plan. At least I have a plan right? I will set aside one hour per day to do a 45 minute workout (the extra time is to include breaks and DVD changing, kid interruptions, etc). I will do the Yoga X every day and the Ab Ripper X every other day. The days I only do Yoga X, I will do that for 45 minutes and the days I do both I will do like I did today 30/15. That's my plan. I know it may sound a bit wimpy for some people but for me it's a mountain to climb.

May 22 through June 30 - another 40 day plan ending July 1st. Don't ask me why - I just need to have a start and finish line for some reason. That will keep me motivated. As for eating, well, that's another plan I'm going to have to come up with. I talked about seasonal eating with one weekly reward. Maybe that will be a good starting point. Looks like my 40 day Survivor Diet Challenge just got upgraded. I don't know if I'll continue to log every day like I have been (this is really time consuming) but I have to admit, it keeps me on track - so we'll see.

I am going to have to create another set of rules for this next wave.

CONCLUSION

The Survivor Diet Challenge was a complete success! I achieved my goal of losing weight, getting healthy and having a tremendous amount of fun and adventure in the process. I learned a lot about myself and a lot about the nearby natural environment. I can honestly say that I did things that I never thought I would find myself doing. I stayed active and busy and engaged the entire time. I never suffered or felt starved or malnourished. All of my previous issues such as headaches, high blood pressure, bloated feeling, gassiness, laziness (ha) – have all but disappeared.

It will be a challenge to maintain this mindset without the guidance of strict rules or a daily log to keep me honest and motivated. Only time will tell how successful the diet really is but a lot of that has to do with the individual and his/her will power. My Survivor Diet Challenge is a jump start to healthiness – a 40 day plan to kick your body and mind into gear. Build a foundation, lose weight, get healthy, learn new skills and then the rest is up to you.

I talked a lot in the first pages of this book about how the body is a machine that, if fed the right fuel, will grow and thrive and heal and learn. If fed the wrong fuel, it will slowly die. Natural, whole foods that grow locally and seasonally are the answer. Reducing obesity is the answer. Extra weight, extra fat, extra toxins and preservatives – these are the poisons that kill our machines. It's so easy and 'convenient' to grab a quick meal of prepared fast food but if you take a step back and look at the big picture, it's just putting you on the fast track to a miserable life and early death.

The Survivor Diet challenges you to find your primitive roots. It's the Paleo Diet on steroids! Do you know why? Because it makes YOU get out there and do the work. Anyone can go to the store and pick out whole, natural foods and purchase them for meals. And yes, that's a great start. But to actually do the things necessary to provide for your meals – that's a whole different ballgame. The doing is also engaging your mind, body and creativity along the journey and these things are just as important to develop as the foods we eat. Knowing where every bit of your food comes from and how to get it is essential.

The Survivor Diet makes you work hard for your food fuel and as such you will learn to appreciate it a lot more. You will learn to waste a lot less. And you will help your machine to heal, grow and prosper.

HEALTHOMETER RESULTS

Day		Time	Weight	Blood Pressure Systolic	Diastolic	Goal - 120	Goal - 80
1	Monday	7:30 AM	190	144	104	120	80
2	Tuesday	7:00 AM	189	138	98	120	80
3	Wednesday	7:00 AM	186	138	100	120	80
4	Thursday	5:00 AM	184	135	104	120	80
5	Friday	7:45 AM	185	130	100	120	80
6	Saturday	7:45 AM	185	132	90	120	80
7	Sunday	9:00 AM	183	135	95	120	80
8	Monday	8:30 AM	185	130	85	120	80
9	Tuesday	7:30 AM	183	128	96	120	80
10	Wednesday	7:00 AM	181	130	98	120	80
11	Thursday	5:00 AM	179	138	102	120	80
12	Friday	5:00 AM	178	130	102	120	80
13	Saturday	8:00 AM	178	130	92	120	80
14	Sunday	8:30 AM	180	128	90	120	80
15	Monday	7:45 AM	179	125	96	120	80
16	Tuesday	7:00 AM	178	128	88	120	80
17	Wednesday	7:00 AM	175	124	98	120	80
18	Thursday	5:00 AM	175	122	94	120	80
19	Friday	6:00 AM	175	130	96	120	80
20	Saturday	9:00 AM	174	132	98	120	80
21	Sunday	8:30 AM	174	120	90	120	80
22	Monday	7:30 AM	179	122	90	120	80
23	Tuesday	7:00 AM	175	120	90	120	80
24	Wednesday	7:00 AM	174	118	88	120	80
25	Thursday	5:00 AM	173	128	100	120	80
26	Friday	7:30 AM	176	130	88	120	80
27	Saturday	8:00 AM	175	120	96	120	80
28	Sunday	8:00 AM	175	118	88	120	80
29	Monday	7:30 AM	175	118	86	120	80
30	Tuesday	7:00 AM	174	122	86	120	80
31	Wednesday	7:00 AM	173	122	88	120	80
32	Thursday	5:00 AM	174	130	100	120	80
33	Friday	8:30 AM	174	128	100	120	80
34	Saturday	7:00 AM	174	128	100	120	80
35	Sunday	6:45 AM	173	130	96	120	80
36	Monday	7:30 AM	172	122	88	120	80
37	Tuesday	7:00 AM	173	126	88	120	80
38	Wednesday	7:00 AM	173	124	84	120	80
39	Thursday	7:00 AM	172	126	88	120	80
40	Friday	8:00 AM	172	124	86	120	80
1 AD	Saturday	9:00 AM	173				
2 AD	Sunday	10:00 AM	181				
3 AD	Monday	11:00 AM	175				
4 AD	Tuesday	12:00 PM	174				
5 AD	Wednesday	1:00 PM	173				

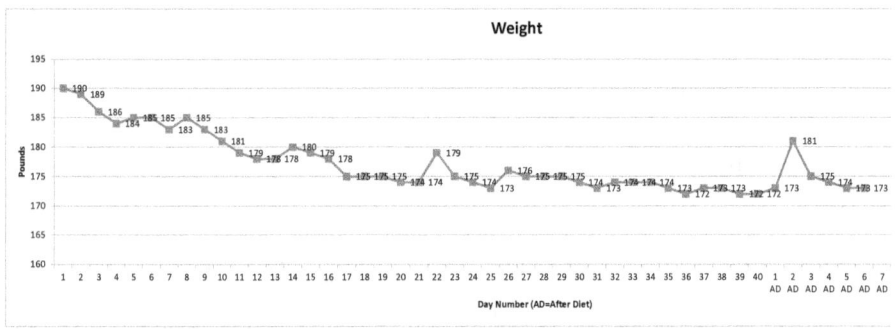

My weight dropped from 190 pounds to 173 pounds during the course of this 40-day program. The most significant drops occurred during the first two weeks and then it was a slower progression to the finish. I attribute that to an initial process of detoxification and then when my body hit my 'ideal' weight around 175 pounds it was unnecessary to lose any more.

At that point in the program I noticed a disappearance of headaches and my sleeping patterns became normal with an elimination of snoring and a noticeable reduction in bodily gas. All very positive results.

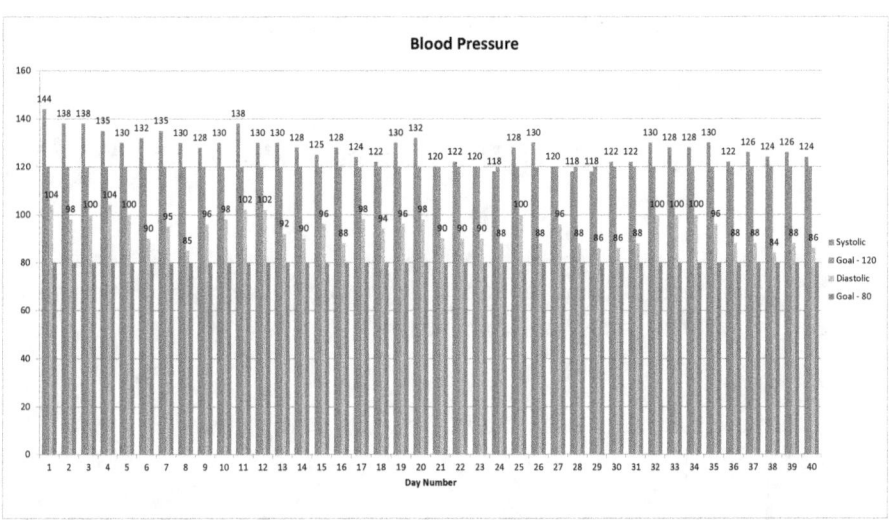

Ideally, blood pressure should be close to 120/80 for a normal healthy individual. Starting near the 140/100 range was a shock to me but after completing my Survivor Diet Challenge my readings were close to normal but very slightly elevated. A huge improvement!

Inspirational Quotes

"It's ok not to know all the answers. It's better to admit our ignorance than to believe answers that might be wrong. Pretending to know everything closes the door to finding out what's really there."
Neil deGrasse Tyson

"Only those who dare to fail greatly can ever achieve greatly."
Robert F. Kennedy

"Stay away from people who belittle your ambition. Small people always do that. The really great people make you feel like you too can be great."
Mark Twain

"The desire for safety stands in the way of every great and noble enterprise."
Cornelius Tacitus

"Unless you try something beyond what you have already mastered, you will never grow."
Ronald E. Osborn

"Failure is the opportunity to begin again more intelligently - keep moving forward."
Henry Ford

"To get what we've never had before, we must do what we have never done before."
Unknown

"Do not live in fear of what the future may hold. Live in the anticipation of the new opportunities that lie ahead."
Unknown

"Whatever the mind can believe and conceive, it can achieve."
Napoleon Hill

"Tis not the meat but the appetite that makes eating a delight."
Sir John Suckling

"The quality of an individual is reflected in the standards they set for themselves."
Ray Kroc

"Don't measure yourself by what you haven't accomplished - but by what you plan to accomplish."
John Wooden (partial)

"Never leave fish."
Gary Peterson

"The difficulties and struggles of today are the price we pay for the successes of tomorrow."
William J. H. Boetcker

"It's the amount that you do over and beyond what's required of you that determines your degree of success."
Unknown

"Whatever the mind can believe and conceive, it can achieve."
Napoleon Hill

"Things turn out the best for the people who make the best of the way things turn out."
John Wooden

"Good judgment comes from experience and experience comes from bad judgment."
Rita Mae Brown

"There are two ways of spreading light - to be the candle or the mirror that reflects it."
Edith Wharton

"From mistakes we learn. From successes - not so much. Keep moving forward."
Meet the Robinsons

"Nothing will ever be attempted if all possible objections must first be overcome."
Samuel Johnson

"A person's manners are a mirror through which he shows his true portrait."
Johann Wolfgang von Goethe

"The spirit, the will to win, the will to endure - these qualities are much more important than the actual events that occur."
Vince Lombardi

"Defeat is not the worst of failures. Not to have tried is the true failure."
George Edward Woodberry

"Not by age, but by capacity is wisdom acquired."
Titus Maccius Plautus

"If you want uncommon success, you must be uncommon."
Unknown

"A ship in port is safe. But that's not what ships were made for. Sail out to sea and do new things."
Grace Hopper

"Expect the best. Prepare for the worst. Capitalize on what comes."
Zig Ziglar

"A storm starts when the first drop starts dropping but when the first drops stop dropping the storm starts stopping."
Dr. Seuss

"To know what to do is wisdom. To know how to do it is skill. But actually doing it tops the other two virtues by far."
Unknown

"Anyone who stops learning is old - whether you're 20 or 80. Anyone who keeps learning keeps young."
Henry Ford

"Success consists of a series of little daily efforts."
Mamie McCullough

"Effort is a commitment to seeing a task through to the end; not just until you get tired of it."
Howard Cate

"Don't wait for extraordinary opportunities. Seize common occasions and make them great."
Orison Swett Marden

"It takes courage to break through barriers and to go places you've never been before."
Anaïs Nin

"We all have possibilities we don't know about. We can do things we don't even dream we can do."
Dale Carnegie

"You may be disappointed if you fail, but you are doomed if you do not try."
Beverly Sills

"Procrastination is the thief of time."
Edward Young

"Success is not final, failure is not fatal: it is the courage to continue that counts."
Winston Churchill

"Believe me, the reward is not so great without the struggle."
Wilma Rudolph

"A person who leaves nothing to chance does very few things wrong. However, he also does very few things."
Unknown

"A great pleasure in life is doing what people say you cannot do."
Walter Bagehot

"Sometimes you have to jump off the cliff and make your wings on the way down."
Ray Bradbury

"Greatness is primarily bravery to escape old ways and customs."
Unknown

"Growth demands a temporary surrender of security."
Gail Sheehy

Doug Peterson's

SURVIVOR
DIET
CHALLENGE

volume 1